MAKING A PLACE
FOR KIDS WITH
DISABILITIES

MAKING A PLACE
FOR KIDS WITH
DISABILITIES

Dale Borman Fink

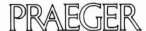

Westport, Connecticut
London

Library of Congress Cataloging-in-Publication Data

Fink, Dale Borman, 1949–
    Making a place for kids with disabilities / Dale Borman Fink.
        p.   cm.
    Includes bibliographical references and index.
    ISBN 0–275–96565–1 (alk. paper)
    1. Handicapped children—Recreation—United States.
    2. Handicapped youth—Recreation—United States.   3. Sports for the
    handicapped—United States.   I. Title.
    GV183.6.F56   2000
    790.1'96—dc21   99–37526

British Library Cataloguing in Publication Data is available.

Library of Congress Catalog Card Number: 99–37526
ISBN: 0–275–96565–1

First published in 2000

Praeger Publishers, 88 Post Road West, Westport, CT 06881
An imprint of Greenwood Publishing Group, Inc.
www.praeger.com

Printed in the United States of America

The paper used in this book complies with the
Permanent Paper Standard issued by the National
Information Standards Organization (Z39.48–1984).

10 9 8 7 6 5 4 3 2 1

Copyright Acknowledgment

The author and publisher gratefully acknowledge permission for use of the following
material:

Excerpts from "Gym I" and "Gym II" by Jeffrey Tolley in *Crossroads,* April 1998. Used
by permission of Jeffrey Tolley and Susan L. Davis.

For Irving L. Fink and Beatrice Borman Fink

Contents

viii   Contents

Preface

You might say my interest in inclusive recreation, sports, and youth programs can be traced to a cup of pine needle tea. Not that I acquired my interest in the topic while I was drinking the stuff but because my sister drank it—or so she claimed—as a teenager, when she attended Flat Rock River Camp.

In 1965, when I was in high school in Indianapolis, Indiana, my mother gave birth to the fifth child in our family. Laurel had what we later learned to call Down Syndrome. At the time, the term used was *mongoloid*. The doctors advised my parents to put the baby in a state institution, because in their opinion she would always be completely dependent, even for her most basic needs. My parents, however, kept their own counsel.

Mom and Dad were Ohio Buckeyes, both of the Jewish variety, who had met when she was a newspaper reporter and he a soldier about to leave for the European theater of World War II. Twenty years into their marriage, they did not envisage themselves as spear carriers for any budding political or social movement, but they could not get comfortable with the idea of abandoning their baby to be a ward of the state, to be cared for (or, more likely, neglected) in one of Indiana's notoriously underfunded residential institutions. Furthermore, the credentialed specialists could not convince them that their daughter was incapable of learning. They wanted to believe that with loving support, she could learn and also that her presence could enrich and add to the life of our family and not simply burden and diminish it, as the experts professed.

Knowing no one facing similar circumstances, they acted alone on these modest but firm convictions. Yet in doing so, Bea and Irving Fink turned out to be part of a whole generation of parents whose choices regarding their offspring with disabilities had a profound impact on the reshaping of our country's laws and attitudes. In the 1970s, the voices of family members of children with disabilities combined with those of adults with physical disabilities, including many returning Vietnam veterans, set in motion waves of change that would wash over our country for more than a generation.

Laurel's development and achievements over the next several decades would more than gratify the hopes my parents held. In 1983, she won a prize in a regional high school art contest for a silk screen of a unicorn she had created in art class. In 1984, she put on a cap and gown and walked with her classmates to the strains of "Pomp and Circumstance." One of the local television news channels covered the event, spotlighting Laurel's achievement as the first person with Down Syndrome in the state's history to receive a high school diploma. They also showed a videotape of her participating in an aerobics class. The message: The conventional wisdom of 1965 had been irrevocably shredded. Laurel and my parents had been part of the shredding.

PINE NEEDLE TEA

Laurel's attendance at a regular overnight camp run by the Indianapolis YMCA when she was 13 years old took place at a time when such an organization was under no legal obligation to enroll a child with a disability (unless it received federal funds). In retrospect, it was the kind of experience that was both contributor to and an effect of the social evolution underway in those pivotal years. New laws had been passed in the 1970s, and the rigid separation of youth with mental disabilities from their peers was slowly breaking down. Children with Down Syndrome and other forms of mental retardation were becoming visible in public schools, yet the vast majority were continuing to be assigned to completely separate classrooms, often in completely separate schools. Still, the climate of change made it possible for my mother to call up the camp director and convince him to enroll Laurel, even though his staff had no experience with children with special needs. Laurel was the camp's first enrollee with a substantial disability of any kind.

This was not only a big step for the camping staff but likewise for Laurel and for my parents. Her schooling up to that point took place strictly in a classroom with other special education students. It was only in our neighborhood that she was accustomed to playing with peers without special needs—usually pairing off with girls several years younger than she.

At camp, there was no one on staff with any specialized training to work with youth with developmental disabilities or even with formal teaching credentials. But with a little information provided by my mother, the camp director and counselors proved willing to take on the challenge. Everything went very smoothly and helped all of us—the camp staff included—to recognize that she could participate in and enjoy activities not specifically designed for youth with special needs.

The camping experience included the usual mix of swimming, hiking the trail, craft activities, eating in the dining hall, singing songs, roasting wieners, and staying with other girls in a cabin. The pleasure and pride she took in her inclusive camping experience left an indelible mark. Whenever any of us are boiling water for a pot of tea in Laurel's presence, she can be counted on to remind us that there is only one kind of tea she drinks: pine needle tea. If anyone asks for further explanation, she will explain that this is what they brewed after a hike at Flat Rock River Camp. Although it was many years in the past, Laurel continues to speak of it with a surprising immediacy.

TAKING AN AUDIT OF MY OWN SUBJECTIVITY

I hope that readers will find me to be a keen, caring, and insightful observer. But a dispassionate objectivity is not one of the assets I bring to this book. The experiences I record in the following pages are filtered through my own past—pine needle tea and all. "Research is not helped by making it appear value free," writes Robert Stake (1995, 95). "It is better to give the reader a good look at the researcher. Often, it is better to leave on the wrappings of advocacy." In a similar vein, Alan Peshkin (1988, 17) suggests that "researchers, notwithstanding their use of quantitative or qualitative methods, their research problem, or their reputation for personal integrity, should systematically identify their subjectivity throughout the course of their research." He recommends what he calls an "audit" of one's own points of special pleading. "I do not thereby exorcise my subjectivity," he explains. "I do, rather, enable myself to manage it" (20).

In offering readers a look at some of my own wrappings, it will help them to see that this book is a result of the "unique configuration" of my "personal qualities joined to the data [I] have collected" (Peshkin 1988, 18). The biases and beliefs I have acquired through my attention to the experiences of my sister are one important aspect of my subjectivity, but not the only one.

Inclusion in After-School Child Care

When I became director of an after-school child care program in 1980, the parent board of directors who hired me were at loggerheads about whether to waive the usual age and grade restrictions in order to permit one parent to enroll his high school–aged son, Lester, with Down Syndrome in our program. I empathized with the parent and advocated strongly for acceptance; the board agreed to make the one-time policy change.

Lester fancied himself a ladies' man and practiced his arts with the women teachers on our staff, all of whom were in their twenties. He enjoyed calling them "sugar" and "honey," and sometimes punctuated his greetings with a hand clasped on the shoulder or a light slap on the buttocks. We tried hard to get Lester to be engaged with the other children in the program but without great success. In retrospect, I see that he resisted greater engagement because he accurately saw the other enrollees as *children* and knew that as an adolescent attending high school, he had moved on to another developmental stage. Overall, this attempt at inclusion satisfied the parent's need for safe, affordable child care in his home neighborhood. But from Lester's point of view, it could not be pronounced a complete success.

Over the next several years, there were more enrollments from families whose children had disabilities, and I believe we did much better for these participants. We accepted two children who used wheelchairs, both of whom also had severe cognitive and language impairments. To make this feasible, we secured support from the school district (which housed, but did not operate, our program) so that we could hire an extra staff person. That Jeremy and Jessica gained a great deal from their attendance at our program was unmistakable. I used to pass many times a day by their school classroom, where they were grouped all day long with peers with similar levels of disability. The teacher was very nice and very competent, but the environment was profoundly sedentary. The only real hustle and bustle was furnished by therapists who paraded in and out of the room all day. Sometimes the service providers outnumbered the students, and all were earnestly performing their various rites of intervention.

In our after-school program, we didn't work on their educational goals. We just gave them the same choices we offered to our other participants: outdoor play, cooking projects, arts, crafts, film watching, or trips to museums, parks, and the municipal swimming pool. Jeremy and Jessica used more language, initiated more social interaction, and showed more enthusiasm during their hours with us than they did during the school day.

We also served without difficulties other children with special needs who did not require any additional staffing: a five-year-old with diabetes (we had to learn to help her regulate her diet and do the finger-prick test for blood sugar level); a 10-year-old with mild hydrocephaly; numerous children who were receiving help for speech and language, motor and vision problems, and mental health and behavior problems.

Gaining a National Perspective

When I left the after-school child care program, it was to join an action research team at Wellesley College in Massachusetts, studying the problems of latchkey children and promoting before- and after-school child care for school-age youngsters. During these years, I surveyed families of school-aged youth with special needs and conducted a national search for program models that addressed the child care needs of school-aged children with disabilities. I visited segregated programs that were established specifically to serve the after-school child care needs of youth with special needs, and inclusive programs (the word used at that time was *integrated*). I interviewed family members of youth with special needs, as well as teachers and caregivers who worked in the programs. This research (Fink 1988) widened my lens and expanded the ideas I had begun developing during my years as a practitioner.

In 1993, I joined the national board of directors of Camp Fire Boys and Girls. One of our nation's traditional youth development organizations, it was founded in 1910 as the Camp Fire Girls, the first nonsectarian organization for girls in the United States. In 1975, the organization amended its charter to become coeducational. My board membership, which continued for four years, added another aspect to my subjectivity. It showed me how our affiliated councils around the country were viewing the changing social and legal landscape that required them to rethink their past practices regarding the participation of children with disabilities. Some councils still operated separate programs for girls and boys with special needs, while others were moving swiftly to make their programs fully inclusive. At a national meeting in Kansas City, Missouri, in 1995, I chaired a panel discussion that provided our adolescent members, board volunteers, and professional staff a forum to explore these changing values and practices.

As a national board member, I was a volunteer, and this experience inclined me to sympathize with any organization that relied on a base of volunteers. I recognized that the loyalties of volunteers could become easily strained if leaders moved too quickly in implementing new practices and policies, regardless of the merit underlying the proposed new policies. Without the homemakers, retirees, wage workers, business owners, and professionals who ran the meetings, recruited the kids, and kept up the organization's name in the community, there would be no programs—inclusive or not.

Graduate School

Simultaneous with the years I was active on the Camp Fire board, I went back to school to earn a Ph.D. in special education. It was in studying the methods of qualitative research that I learned about the importance of informing readers of the sources of my subjectivity, as I am now doing. I also learned that one of my tasks was to familiarize myself with relevant work produced by other authors. Instead of abstracting this work under the rubric of a separate "literature review," I have incorporated references to published literature throughout the chapters that follow, using them wherever they are most relevant to the story I am telling.

SEEKING TO UNDERSTAND MULTIPLE PERSPECTIVES

My interest in inclusion in community-based programs for youth, then, had its origins in my family life. I experienced pain at the barriers my sister faced and vicarious pleasure in her successful adventures, such as her attendance at Flat Rock River Camp. My interest and knowledge were enlarged and my biases further shaped by my experiences as a program supervisor serving youth with and without disabilities in an after-school child care program. In my subsequent career as a researcher, I was able to compare my own experiences as a practitioner with those of other school-age program providers in Texas, California, Wisconsin,

New York, Vermont, the province of Alberta (in Canada), and a variety of other places. My role as a volunteer member of the board of a national youth development organization added another layer to my knowledge and my subjectivity. Finally, my doctoral training gave me new tools to discipline and organize my continuing inquiries into this subject.

The increasing presence of students with disabilities in regular school classrooms has received a great deal of attention in recent years from researchers, parents, and practitioners. But the lives of youngsters with disabilities do not end when they exit their classrooms, and their participation in a wide variety of youth programs and recreational settings is becoming a fact of life in many communities. Yet this latter subject has drawn little focused attention from scholars, journalists, or even the family members of the participants. I saw that a descriptive study, delineating how inclusive participation was evolving in a single community, could fill an important gap in the published literature. At the same time, it would take advantage of my own history.

Denzin (1989, 25) states that "Unlike the positivists, who separate themselves from the worlds they study, the interpretivists participate in the social world so as to understand and express more effectively its emergent properties and features." This is what I set out to do: To inhabit the ball fields, meeting halls, and drop-in centers where children with and without disabilities congregated and recreated during their hours outside school, in one midwestern town.

To whom would I need to bring an empathetic ear in order to conduct the kind of study I proposed? Family members of children with disabilities, program administrators, volunteers in recreation and youth development programs, as well as children. The path I had walked had given me experience in each of those roles.

Acknowledgments

Tim Nugent, director of rehabilitation services at the University of Illinois, organized the first wheelchair basketball tournament in the United States in Galesburg, Illinois, in 1949 (DePauw and Gavron 1995, 59). More than 45 years later, he was helping Erica, whose Brownie troop experiences I profile in Chapter 6, to get the therapeutic services she needed. It was Erica's grandmother who informed me about this retired professor whom she knew to be a pioneer in recreation for people with disabilities. And thus do the trails between what we call the "world of research" and the "world of practice" lead back and forth in unpredictable ways.

I could not have conducted the research for this book without the cooperation of Leonard Schmidt, Bob Nuchols, Ruth Kulmala, Betty Gregg, Susan Jean, and Mike and Di Ostrander. I am also grateful for the assistance provided by Chris and Ken Bilek, Deborah Bruns, Sam Burdette, Mary Coash, Karen Comeau, Deanna Eddy, Stephanie Eddy, Vickie and Richard Eichenlaub, Sandy Heins, Karla Hill, Pam and Paulette Hurd, Laura Lieb, Robert and Sandra Lindsay, Sandy McAuley, Beckie Neal, Ron Oser, Janie Hughes-Oser, Mark and Debra Owen, Danita Perkins, Teri Post, T. C. Randolph, Marcia Roberts, Mary Sarbaugh, Deborah Schmidt, William Shields, and Wanda White.

I left the community I called Wabash with very fond feelings, owing to the courtesy and warmth that so many people there extended to me.

Thanks to all the girls named Ashley (there were so many of them!) and all the other youngsters whom I cannot name for reasons of confidentiality.

I was earning a Ph.D. at the University of Illinois at Urbana-Champaign when I conducted the research for this book. I benefited from having as my advisor Susan Fowler, a truly gifted teacher. I was instructed in qualitative research methods by the very best: Robert Stake (my dissertation advisor), Liora Bresler, and Alan Peshkin. Adelle Renzaglia, Bob Henderson, Jeanette McCollum, Mickie Ostrosky, and Tess Bennett were some of the other faculty who made the special education department an intellectually vibrant, socially supportive, and community-minded place.

Thanks to Jeffrey Tolley and Susan Davis for permission to reprint two poems, and to John Harney for believing in the importance of this book. At various stages of the writing, I received important editorial comments from Sarah Hadden, Beatrice Borman Fink, Helen Zimmerberg, and Randall Miller, M.D.

When I was working on my dissertation, I used to call up Betty Zimmerberg and read drafts of chapters to her out loud over the phone. When she came to visit, we drove around Wabash, and I showed her the location of the baseball diamonds, the Karate School, the trailer parks, and the Chinese buffet. She remains my most trusted literary advisor, and in 1998 we began writing a new book together. The first chapter was called "Our Wedding."

Introduction: Inclusive Recreation and Sports Enter the Mainstream

When Casey Martin sank a 25-foot putt to win a dramatic playoff in Cincinnati, Ohio, on June 8, 1998, and qualify for the U.S. Open, the first person to congratulate him was his caddy. The second was 11-year-old Will Ard, a Cincinnati resident whose mother had brought him to watch the tournament. Why? Because the youngster and the professional each lived with the same congenital circulatory problem, Klippel-Trénaunay-Weber syndrome. "Will likes to play baseball," Will's mother told *New York Times* reporter Clifton Brown. "We feel there's been a little prejudice in the Little League toward him. It's pretty upsetting. I wanted him to see Casey, to see what he can accomplish" (8 June 1998, C-1).

Martin had quickly become nationally visible when he filed a lawsuit under the provisions of the Americans with Disabilities Act (ADA). "Disabled Pro Golfer Fights No-cart Rule," the *Washington Post* announced to its readers on page one (Steve Harrison, 10 December 1997). A month later, *USA Today* ran a long background piece on the front of its sports section called "Pro Golfer Rides Out Storm" (Harry Blauvelt, 7 January 1998). Articles followed in dozens of local newspapers across the country in both sports and news pages.

It was fitting that an 11-year-old with special needs was present to cheer for Martin on the occasion of his triumph in Cincinnati. For in their prominent reportage of the story of golfer Casey Martin, newspapers and broadcasters across the United States had brought into the mainstream of national consciousness a discussion that had previously been taking place at Boy Scout jamborees and in Brownie troops, among recreation professionals and camp directors, and on the soccer and baseball fields of cities and towns across America. The nub of the discussion was this: If we are no longer excluding kids with disabilities from the activities enjoyed by their more typically developing peers, then what new obligations do we take on in order to make a place for them?

It was paradoxical that Martin was the person who brought this issue into the public arena. Up to this point, Martin's had been an American success story, his physical impairment a footnote that had neither handicapped his learning nor sidelined him from his favorite sport. He attended Stanford, one of the premier universities in the country, and there he met all academic expectations while captaining the golf team to an NCAA championship in 1994.

However, Klippel-Trénaunay-Weber syndrome was an adversary that would never be defeated. It caused the blood flowing to his right leg to pool and throb, and the leg to swell. It required him to use pain medication daily and to wrap the leg in support hose all day and night, removing the wrap only when he showered (Blauvelt, "Golfer Rides Out Storm"). He was able to achieve success while at Stanford because the decision makers in collegiate golf allowed him to use a motorized cart at times when he needed it.

The Professional Golf Association declined to oblige him in similar fashion, and his condition was worsening. At age 25, when he realized he could not continue walking the course in pain, it was to the ADA, passed in 1990, that Casey Martin was able to turn for legal redress. Absent accommodations for his disability, he would be unable to use his gifts and pursue his aspirations. He would have to forfeit his career.

CALIFORNIA BOY WANTED TO PLAY BASEBALL

The encounter between Casey Martin and a young fan illustrated that it was only Martin's visibility, owing to his professional-level talent, that made his circumstances exceptional. His desire to be a full-fledged participant resonated not only with Will Ard but also with tens of thousands of other youngsters across the country with physical, medical, emotional, or mental impairments.

Unfortunately, the resistance that Martin confronted when he sought permission to ride the golf course in a cart was also familiar to some kids who had tried to join in with the recreational activities of their peers. Geoffrey Shultz, an 11-year-old with cerebral palsy, wanted to play competitive baseball in a summer league in Hemet, California, in 1994. He had previously played two years in tee-ball, where he had experienced no problems. At age 11, his parents requested that he be allowed to play in the 9 and 10-year-old division, down one level from others his age, so that he could more easily face a pitched ball for the first time. He had intended to bat with one arm while supporting himself with a crutch and then use both crutches to run the basepaths.[1]

The league officials, after consulting with the governing body of Pony Baseball Inc., did not allow his family to register him to play down. When Geoffrey's father then tried to sign him up for a regular 11-and 12-year-old team, they also denied that request. In doing so, they cited the liability they would face in the event Geoffrey became injured. They also stated to the parents that if he played, he might embarrass himself.

Geoffrey's family went to federal court on his behalf, and they won. U.S. District Court Judge Consuelo B. Marshall found that the local baseball league and Pony Baseball were in violation of the ADA as well as two California laws (*Geoffrey Shultz v. Hemet Youth Pony League, Inc., Don Nelson; David Dekonty; and Does 1 through 10 and related counteractions*, 943 F.Supp.1222). The judge found that the defendants had excluded Geoffrey "on the basis of assumed and unsubstantiated concerns of a possible risk of harm." In a subsequent ruling, the judge ordered the defendants to pay the family $15,000 in damages.[2] This story did not enjoy the kind of national spotlight drawn three years later by the Martin case, but it illuminated the fact that barriers to addressing individual differences existed for youth seeking recreational sports opportunities and not just for aspiring professional athletes.

Like Shultz before him, Martin too was successful in court. As described in the *Washington Post* on December 2, 1997 (E-2), he first obtained a restraining order from a federal magistrate, which allowed him to use his cart during a qualifying tour in December 1997. Using the cart, he then played well enough to qualify for the Nike Tour, one step down in competition level from the PGA Tour (Harrison, "Golfer Fights Rule"). Martin then won a further favorable ruling from a federal district judge who granted him permission to use his cart during the Nike Tour, a story the *New York Times* emblazoned on its front page rather than its sports section (Marcia Chambers, "Judge Says Disabled Golfer May Use Cart on Pro Tour," 12 February 1998). While the PGA appealed that decision, the United States Golf Association agreed to let him use a cart for the qualifying round and (if he qualified) for play in the U.S. Open, although it was not a party to the previous ruling (*New York Times*, 31 March 1998, C-7). That set the stage for his dramatic victory in Cincinnati.

HEROES OF PAST NEEDED NO ACCOMMODATIONS?

In the wake of the publicity about the case, strong opinions were expressed, and many were unsympathetic to Martin. His request to have his individual needs addressed by the use of a motorized cart were contrasted to memories of Ben Hogan, a golfer of legendary repute, who was injured in a car crash in 1949. Although he had trouble walking after that, he still managed to win major tournaments. In 1953, after winning the Masters, U.S. Open, and British Open, Hogan skipped the PGA Championship because of weariness. Thus he forfeited the chance to become the first golfer ever to win all four spurs of golf's "Grand Slam" (Harrison, "Golfer Fights Rule").

The inference from such a precedent is that the participant with special needs is obliged to adapt himself to the standard rules and procedures, not the other way around. A second inference might be that the proud heroes of the past would never expect anyone to accommodate their individual needs: They succeeded (or failed) strictly on their own capacities. Of course, one could also look back with a different perspective, as does Tom Sullivan, a former network television correspondent who is also blind and a golfer. "Golf was denied many more opportunities to see this great man [Hogan] play because . . . well, because he was not allowed to use a cart" ("My Turn; A Question of Fair Play," *Newsweek*, 16 February 1998, 16).

Regardless of the ultimate disposition of the case or the trajectory of his career,[3] the publicity surrounding Casey Martin's attempt to have his individual needs acknowledged and addressed gave large numbers of people their first opportunity to ponder and reconsider the way our society has thought about this issue. For all the Ben Hogans who participated and succeeded (at least, some of the time) without any acknowledgment of their individual differences or needs, how many others dropped out of the competition? How many potentially gifted athletes never participated at all? The recognition of Martin's right to golf with the aid of a cart was an important link in a chain that extended back across many years and many different arenas.

A LOOK BACK

At the first Special Olympics in 1968, doctors warned Eunice Kennedy Shriver, the creator of the event, that "the participants' fragile hearts might not withstand a run of more than 400 meters" (Shapiro 1991, 11). Twenty-five years later, the International Special Olympics was sponsoring half-marathons (13.1 miles), and athletes with mental disabilities from across the globe were running them. Not only had an enormous enlargement of opportunities for young people and adults with special needs taken place during a single generation, but in that same short period of years, there had been an astonishing shift in what passed as "expert opinion."

Convincing society that they were mentally, physically, and emotionally capable of taking on the same kinds of challenges that their more typically developing peers enjoyed was one hurdle that youngsters and adults with various kinds of disabilities had to clear. Given a league of their own, as it were, in which to prepare themselves and prove their abilities, they had jumped over the bar with room to spare.

But the next hurdle was in some ways more vexing. Predominant practice well into the 1970s was based on the belief that young people with disabilities—if they were allowed to participate at all—would benefit more from having their own separate times in the pool, on the field, attending the dancing lesson, the karate class, or the summer camp. How and when could they (at least, the ones who preferred this option) be viewed as no longer in need of a league of their own? What would it take for them to be viewed as team members, troop members, club members, participants entitled to join in the same community-based programs that appealed to their neighbors and siblings who had no identified special needs?

Civil Rights and Special Education Laws

Discrimination against persons with disabilities was prohibited in federally funded programs by Section 504 of the Rehabilitation Act of 1973. This was a milestone in the civil rights of persons with disabilities in the United States. Programs receiving funds from the federal government were required to make reasonable accommodations in order that everyone "otherwise qualified" might gain access and have an opportunity to participate.

Two years later, every person in the United States from ages 5 to 21 who had disabilities or special learning needs became entitled for the first time, by Public Law 94–142, (later renamed the Individuals with Disabilities Education Act, or IDEA) to an appropriate public education, individualized to address her or his specific learning goals. As part of that law, parents were given an unprecedented role in shaping and approving the plans proposed by educators. The educational programs were to be delivered in the "least restrictive environment," an expression whose interpretation was a continuing point of contention a quarter century later but which tilted toward the education of students who had disabilities in the classrooms where they would be if they had no special needs.

ADA Lays Foundation for Expanded Participation

In the 1990s, civil rights for persons with disabilities were dramatically advanced—at least on paper—by the passage of the Americans with Disabilities Act (1990), which carried by an overwhelming bipartisan consensus in both houses of Congress. It outlawed discrimination in employment, state and municipal government, public accommodations, transportation, telecommunications, and a range of other arenas. This was a signal for a new level of participation for Americans who had disabilities. While Section 504 (1973) had restricted discrimination in programs that received federal dollars, the new law prohibited discrimination in a wide range of programs and activities, irrespective of the presence or absence of federal funds. While the IDEA guaranteed children with special learning needs a right to appropriate schooling, the new law ensured that they could participate in any program or activity that was open to other members of the public, and they could have their individual needs reasonably accommodated. No longer could they be shunted into special programs for "special" or "exceptional" persons—unless that was their preference. Youth and recreation programs were nearly all subject to Section 504, the ADA, or both. They were subject to the former if they were recipients of federal dollars and to the latter as entities of state or municipal government (e.g., local park departments) or as public accommodations.

Organizations that were formerly involved with the promotion of segregated services for those with disabilities reversed course and became part of the push for inclusion. The Delegate Body of the Arc (formerly the Association for Retarded Citizens) adopted a position statement in 1992 (xix) strongly endorsing "Inclusive Recreation and

Leisure." The resolution called on "organizations currently providing segregated recreation and leisure activities to develop inclusive options" and called inclusive recreation and leisure "an essential component of a quality life for people with mental retardation." Special Olympics began an initiative called Unified Sports in which they recruited teams made up of only 50 percent of athletes with mental disabilities and 50 percent of athletes of comparable age and ability with no special needs.

ATTITUDES AS IMPORTANT AS LAWS

In the league where Geoffrey Shultz had wanted to play in Hemet, California, the vast majority of the other players and their parents voiced support for his right to participate, crutches and all, his mother told me. The coaches even took a vote in favor of letting him join a team.[4] It was only the governing board of the local league and its national sanctioning body that blocked his participation.

The active support Geoffrey received from other families, coaches, and peers was good news, not only for this one boy and his family but for others across the country. To fully participate, children with disabilities needed not only the support of changed laws and practices but also the understanding of community members.

Making adaptations for those with disabilities was often imagined to be a costly proposition. Yet, in many cases, what was required was not a new architectural design—not even a motorized golf cart. What was needed was personal empathy. Justice Brennan wrote in a 1987 Supreme Court decision, "society's accumulated myths and fears about disability and disease are as handicapping as are the physical limitations that flow from actual impairment" (*School board of Nassau County v Arline*, 107 S. Ct. 1123, 1987).

Jeffrey Tolley, a young adult in his early twenties, who loved to play basketball, found that the teenagers, whom he tried to join in with at his neighborhood gym in North Carolina, were unreceptive. The problem was not one of administrative exclusion, such as Geoffrey Shultz had faced, but of being stigmatized and unwanted. Luckily for him, he met a poet named Susan Davis who got him started writing poetry in a workshop.[5] One day he crafted this poem and asked her to type it up immediately so he could post it on the recreation center bulletin board:

Gym I
I feel sad
because nobody over there like me
because I'm like this
you know, handicapped.
They're human beings. They're not like us
you know, over here.
They can talk right,
not me.
They're big.
I'm small.
I say
"I can touch the rim."
They say, "No you can not!"
But you know I did.
I proved to myself I can touch the rim.
They say, "Hey boy!"
They call me boy.
Those teenagers don't like me.
One guy said "I don't want to play with you.
You're too ugly."
They don't feel like I'm one of them.
I'm not a human being.
I don't talk right,
and they don't want to be my friend.

He posted the poem and apparently the other participants read it with interest. Just a few days later, Tolley returned to Ms. Davis's class and drafted a sequel to the first poem.

Gym II
All the guys at the gym
said they were sorry.
They didn't know I was
you know what
retarded.
I showed them the poem
and they said they understood.
They said "Come and play with me!"
And I ran down the court with them,
and I forgave them.

PARTICIPATION OF THOSE WITH DISABILITIES NOT YET FULLY SETTLED

In the United States at the dawn of the new millennium, there was a growing expectation, underscored by the passage of laws, especially the Americans with Disabilities Act, that children and adults with disabilities should no longer be automatically excluded, as they once would have been, from a wide range of activities. But how, exactly, were they supposed to fit in with their various medical, cognitive, physical, behavioral, or other limitations? It was during this period of flux, in which practices were changing and operators of community-based sports, youth, and recreational programs were seeing increasing numbers of kids with disabilities wanting to participate, that the Martin case came along to challenge the assumptions of the past and galvanize public discussion of these important issues. The Martin and Shultz cases illustrated that the readiness of organizations sponsoring activities to permit full participation of those with disabilities was not yet a fully settled matter. This was true whether you were an accomplished, professional-level athlete or a preadolescent wanting to play for fun. Jeffrey Tolley's experience showed that full acceptance was not a given, even when the law and organizational practices were on your side.

"I don't want to be a poster child. I just want to play golf," was Casey Martin's comment about the notoriety his case received (Blauvelt, "Golfer Rides Out Storm"). Likewise, Jeffrey Tolley never intended to become a poet—he just wanted to play basketball.

Neither lawsuits nor poetry form any part of the remainder of the narrative of this book, which unfolds in a relatively small community in the American Midwest. Yet I encountered at times there the same questions, uncertainties, and fears that led to the pleadings—both legal and poetic—with which readers are now acquainted.

If you will find yourself a seat on the bleachers, let us see what we can learn.

1

Lindy's Wish

Lindy* was a trim, energetic child whose developmental delays and health problems were well masked by her dazzling smile and socially appropriate manners. To meet her, you wouldn't guess that she had undergone heart surgery three times and hip surgery once. You would notice a few things, though. She wore glasses and had a hard time pronouncing words with the *r* sound in them. And there were those times she suited up with her softball team but sat on the bench the entire game, because the volatility of her sugar levels was depleting her energy. When each game ended, she lined up with her teammates to receive the snack from that game's designated parent volunteer—but then handed the cookie, juice pop, or other treat to her sister and got a different snack from her mom, one customized to her restricted diet.

On the field, she did pretty well, rotating through all the positions like her teammates and running with a somewhat awkward gait. While she was playing first base one evening, she stuck out her glove and serendipitously snagged a line drive. She looked astonished, but no more so than most of her teammates would have been. "If she hadn't been so surprised, she probably could have stepped on the base and made it a double play!" her dad said.

---

* Names of persons and communities are fictionalized to protect their privacy and anonymity.

There was that one time she was the first-base runner, and the next batter launched a pretty good hit. Lindy was so excited she ran from first to second, then right up through the pitcher's mound to home. "As she crossed home plate, the other team was like, 'where did she come from?'" her dad chuckled. The umpire waved her back to do it correctly. This sort of miscue didn't bother her teammates or the fans, except for that one grandma who made disparaging remarks one time, not knowing the child's parents were nearby on the bleachers. But her objection had as much to do with the fact that Lindy was African American as with her limitations as a ball player. Anyway, the parents only had to hear such "ugly words" once. "Other parents straightened her out," Lindy's mother commented. "And I don't mean just one or two. It was like the whole crowd stood up to her."

Most people outside the family didn't know why she stopped playing ball in the Wabash Park and Recreation Department (WPRD) league after age nine. The officials of the WPRD said Lindy was getting too tall to play in the coach-pitched league with the seven- and eight-year-olds, but she wasn't physically capable of competing with the girls her own age.

That prompted the family to look into Special Olympics for the first time, although they had to drive her 20 minutes farther, to another town, for that. They inquired first about her playing softball in Special Olympics but learned she was too young. At her age, she was eligible only for their track and field program, so she joined that instead.

Her parents said she found it very exciting. In contrast to her inclusive experiences in her home community, there were a great many older youth and adults involved. It gave her a real charge to compete as an equal against them. Sometimes, they reported, she would take the hand of a less athletically inclined adult competitor and run part way around the track with him or her. She earned her way to the state finals three times, and in her last competition, she won gold medals in both the 50-yard dash and the running long jump.

Special Olympics gave her an avenue to socialize and compete with other persons with mental disabilities. Meanwhile, she continued to be active in Junior Girl Scouts and also in a bowling league in her own community of Wabash. In these two activities, there were no other kids with disabilities. Her average bowling score was 55, not counting the lower scores she obtained while bowling from a wheelchair following her hip surgery.

As she entered the final seasons of her life, the Make-A-Wish Foundation offered to send her and a parent anywhere she wanted. Wabash was within driving distance of St. Louis, and because she had been to several St. Louis Cardinal baseball games already, you might have thought she would have picked Disney World or another destination more heavily advertised as a youngster's nirvana. But she knew what she liked most in the world, and her parents are still proud to display the photographs of their happy girl posing with future Hall of Famer short-stop Ozzie Smith, her favorite of all the players. Lindy died before that year ended, her energy strong all the way to the end, says her mother, but her heart no longer able to do its work. She was 12 years old.

A WINDOW ONTO INCLUSION IN RECREATIONAL SETTINGS

It was just a few months after Lindy's passing that I began to study the youth and recreation programs of a midwestern town, which I called Wabash. It was a community of about 14,000 people, sur-rounded by smaller farming-oriented towns. Her parents were kind enough to meet with me and share their photographs and stories, al-though their grieving was not yet complete. Lindy's mom had left her position as a nurse one day before Lindy died, and she had not yet re-turned to her job when I met her. Although I never met Lindy, her ex-periences helped me to frame the issues that I wanted to explore.

Community Attitudes toward Youth with Special Needs

It was bracing to hear about the general acceptance of one bright-eyed girl by peers, coaches, and the broader community—at least as seen through the eyes of her parents. I hoped to find out how comfort-able the people in Wabash generally were with the presence of children with special needs in youth programs or recreational settings. I won-dered if there was a connection between acceptance (or discomfort) with youth who had disabilities in recreational settings and the extent to which people had contact with the same children in their neighbor-hood schools.

In addition to getting a fix on the attitudes of individual families and the community at large, I hoped to learn whether public agencies and private organizations had adopted policies or practices to ensure equal access to or to address the individual needs of youth with disabilities. Did paid recreation staff and volunteer leaders in youth programs look with favor on the increasing participation of youngsters with special needs? Or did they resist this development?

Segregated Options, Inclusive Options

Lindy spent most of her school time in a segregated class with other special education students. Outside of school, she engaged in softball, bowling, and Girl Scouts with groups consisting of typically developing peers from the Wabash community. As a child with disabilities, Lindy had other options as well: In the nearby city of Brewster, a division of the municipal park department devoted to "special recreation" administered a variety of activities geared exclusively to children and adults with disabilities,[1] including the Special Olympics and a summer camp. I was interested in learning what parents and children thought about these different options and whether other families had the same comfort level as Lindy's mom and dad in encouraging their children to participate in both inclusive and specialized programming. If families did use one type of programming and not the other, would this be on account of their philosophy and values, or did it come down to more practical factors, such as scheduling, cost, and transportation?

Level of Commitment Expected of Family

One or both of Lindy's parents were present any time she participated in any of the inclusive activities mentioned. They did not consider it a burden, as both parents had been active as volunteer leaders in Girl Scouts and bowling when Lindy's older siblings (who had no disabilities) were of school age. Lindy's Tee-ball and softball experiences—so long as they lasted—did not rely on having a parent as a coach but did require that one of them be present for practices as well as games. I hoped to learn whether other parents had to be similarly available as volunteers, or standing by in case they were needed, to ensure equal access to the recreational settings of Wabash.

Keeping Children with Their Own Age Groups—or Not

Advocates for inclusion generally concur that persons with special needs ought to be learning, working, or enjoying leisure and recreation with others of the same stage of development (Moon 1994; Rynders and Schleien 1991), but they are not as explicit about whether they should be assigned with others of their own exact age, as they would if they had no disabilities. Lindy's career in the WPRD softball league was extended for one year by allowing her to play with seven- and eight-year-olds when she had already turned nine. Then, when she was 10 to 12 years old, she participated in Special Olympics with athletes who were adults—way beyond her stage of development—as well as other participants her own age. Her story raised questions in my mind that I wanted to explore with other families and program operators in the community of Wabash. How important was it to keep youth with disabilities in the same age groupings that applied to others? Were there times when a child or adolescent with special needs could benefit from participation in recreational activities with younger or older youth, or even with participants at a different developmental stage of life?

Modifying Equipment, Routines, or Activities

Lindy's parents did not identify any instances in which they expected rules, routines, or other aspects of the activities to be adapted or modified by program leaders in order to ensure their daughter's ability to participate. The only modifications that they mentioned were the ones that they could take care of on their own. This included bringing snacks to the Tee-ball or softball game and offering them to Lindy as an alternative to the ones that other parents distributed. It also included keeping the coach informed about her condition and sometimes requesting him to keep her on the bench when she was weak, due to her brittle diabetes.

A few parents, on their own initiative, having observed her parents giving Lindy a separate snack, asked about Lindy's diet. When it was their turn, they furnished snacks for the whole team that were appropriate for Lindy to eat. This came as a pleasant surprise to Lindy's parents. It exceeded their expectations about what others should do to make accommodations for their daughter.

I wondered if other Wabash families had the same idea as Lindy's mom—that coaches and other youth leaders "should just go on doing what they ordinarily did, and it was my job to pick up the slack for her individual needs." Would this mirror the beliefs of the coaches, troop leaders, or recreation professionals (i.e., would they, too, expect the parents to take the responsibility for helping to implement modified forms of participation for those who needed it)? Or would they take some of this responsibility on their own shoulders?

In planning or implementing modified forms of participation, how much communication would take place between parents and program leaders? Would parents offer suggestions about how to manage their children's behavior, or how to individualize activities for them? Would leaders ask permission, or seek advice from parents, when they wanted to do things differently?

Beyond Acceptance—to Social Interaction and Friendship?

Lindy's teammates "would direct her where she belonged, took her under their wing" during the softball games, Lindy's mom said. But when I asked whether the social interaction that took place during games ever extended to the formation of real friendships, the answer was no. "She was invited to birthday parties once or twice. Parents worried about her medical needs, and I can't say I blamed them." To what extent would that experience, and that perspective, be echoed by others from the same community? When children with special needs became participants in community-based youth programs and recreational settings, did this lead to positive social interactions—even friendships—with more typically developing peers?

LINDY'S WISH—AND MINE

Schleien, McAvoy, Lais, and Rynders (1993, 6) describe inclusion (using the term of art that was popular a few years earlier, *integration*), as consisting of two aspects.

Integration, whether educational, political, recreational, or social, is both a *goal* and a *process*. The goal is to ensure that persons with disabilities are (a) accepted as members of the community, (b) permitted to participate in activities enjoyed by other members of society, and (c) able to participate in the activities alongside peers without disabilities. The process of facilitating integration is not an easy one. It requires social as well as physical integration before relationships can be formed that support mutual benefits and outcomes.

As I looked at each activity and arena in which youth, with and without disabilities, participated in Wabash, I looked for evidence that individuals were, or were not alert to the goal of inclusion, the process of inclusion, or both.

Lindy's wish was to visit with her favorite baseball players and watch them in action one more time; mine was to make use of the insights available from careful attention to Lindy's story. If readers from other communities are able to see in the youth, the families, the volunteers and community members of this case study issues and practices that they wish to examine anew, then let them continue the dialogue—at their camps, in their groups and troops and recreation centers, as well as in other articles and books. That would be the finest way to recognize both Lindy's wish and mine, and a fitting way to honor the people of the town I call Wabash.

2

Embarking on a Qualitative
Case Study

The methods of qualitative inquiry, such as interviews, participant observation, and the review of documents or archives, lent themselves to answering the kinds of questions I had decided to ask. Moreover, these were the kinds of research activities that would most capitalize on the empathy I felt as a family member of a person with developmental disabilities, a former program administrator, and an experienced youth program volunteer. What also appealed to me about doing this kind of research was the nature of the writing that would be required. Few kinds of research left as much room for artfulness in the presentation of results. I looked forward to weaving together field notes, interview excerpts, and readings of related studies into a coherent whole that would be meaningful and engaging to readers, most of whom I assumed would not have an academic or research background.

Yet neither my subject nor the protocols of qualitative research compelled me to focus this study on a single community. To opt for a case study of a single community was to seek the most in-depth, richly contextualized understanding possible. Within a single community, one could probe deeply into the issues and dynamics that supported or inhibited the participation of youth with special needs in various recreational arenas. One could visit and become familiar with the facilities and the people who delivered the programs. Which of the available options (if any) attracted youth with disabilities and their families? On what basis did the parents and children make decisions to join up, to continue, or to drop out of activities? Were there any key leaders to whom parents turned for help? Were policies or practices evolving from one year to another? What were the attitudes of people in the broader community about persons with disabilities?

My hope was to paint a landscape for readers and show them what practices were evolving and what questions, issues, and problems were arising in this one community. Readers could then judge for themselves the relevance of what they saw in this community to the landscapes in which they spent their own lives. They could apply the lessons of this case study (or not) in a process that Stake (1978, 6–7) called "naturalistic generalization."

Naturalistic generalizations develop within a person as a product of experience. They derive from the tacit knowledge of how things are, why they are, how people feel about them, and how these things are likely to be later or in other places with which this person is familiar. They seldom take the form of predictions but lead regularly to expectation. . . . It is the legitimate aim of many scholarly studies to discover or validate laws. But the aim of the practical arts is to get things done. The better generalizations often are those more parochial, those more personal. . . . As readers recognize essential similarities to cases of interest to them, they establish the basis for naturalistic generalization.

In this study, the case was more than a single individual, event, or site. It was the town I named Wabash, a community of 14,000 people. I set out to learn as much as possible about this one community's experience with inclusion of youth with special needs in (or their absence from) sports, youth programs, and recreational settings. Yet in order to do that, I could not confine my lens only to that community and to its present circumstances. I had to familiarize myself with events that took place far away from Wabash and long before the study began. Wabash was part of a nation, and I had to understand how national trends left their imprint on the people and places I visited. "Data records are constructed in and of the local context, but those records cannot be interpreted without reference to their larger milieu" (Graue and Walsh 1995, 140).

I had set foot in Wabash only once before I began to study it. In this chapter, I recount the story behind the story; that is, the research process that produced this book.

WHY I CHOSE WABASH

There were two reasons why I did not choose to conduct a case study in Brewster, the community in which I lived. First, with a population close to 100,000, the number of recreational options for youth with and without special needs was too large and multifaceted to be manageable without access to an entire team of researchers. Second, its recreation department included a separate division to serve children and adults with disabilities. I preferred to study a place where parents' decisions about their children's participation (or nonparticipation) in the recreational arena would mostly revolve around the activities organized for children without special needs. Therefore, I needed to find a smaller community within easy driving distance of Brewster.

My informants during this preliminary round of the inquiry included professors at the state university, Cooperative Extension agents in two counties, and several parents of children with special needs who were personally or professionally active as advocates for their own and other people's children with disabilities. Initial telephone calls yielded three possible nearby venues—Wabash, St. Charles, and Jefferson City—where I could find youth with disabilities participating in recreational settings. I conducted interviews with potential key informants in each of these three communities.

St. Charles had a 4-H club in which several children with special needs had been learning to groom and ride horses. It sounded like a delightful venue for observations, if possibly treacherous for a researcher under chiropractic care for back problems. Unfortunately, outside of this one club, it appeared that I would find few if any other youth with disabilities who were involved in recreational or youth programs in St. Charles.

In Jefferson City, I ascertained that there were a sufficient number of children with special needs active in local programs to make conducting the study there a possibility. I also identified some parents receptive to my inquiry, and it appeared that with their help, I could readily identify others. With respect to Wabash, I came to the same conclusion. At this point, I faced the choice to go forward with the study either in Jefferson City or in Wabash. In *The Art of Case Study Research*, Robert Stake (1995, 4) asks, "How shall cases be selected? The first criterion should be to maximize what we can learn. Given our purposes, which cases are likely to lead us to understandings, to assertions, perhaps even to modifying of generalizations? . . . If we can, we need to pick cases which are easy to get to and hospitable to our inquiry, perhaps for which a prospective informant can be identified and with actors (the people studied) willing to comment on certain draft materials."

Three aspects distinguished Wabash from Jefferson City at the time I had to make the decision: (a) Youth with more substantial disabilities were participating in recreational programs in Wabash; (b) Jefferson City was one of the more affluent in the county, whereas Wabash contained a greater degree of racial and cultural diversity and a higher level of poverty; (c) My initial contact in Wabash, a woman named Rosemary, had an exceptional range of contacts both with parents of youth with disabilities and with youth programs. I knew no one with a comparable network in Jefferson City.

Each of these reasons carried weight, and together they added up to what I considered sound reasons for selecting Wabash as my case study community. Once that decision was made, the real work began.

MY APPROACH TO THE RESEARCH

In their book, *Qualitative Research for Education*, authors Bogdan and Biklen (1992, 29–32) identify five defining features of qualitative research methodology: (1) "Qualitative research has the natural setting as the direct source of data and the researcher is the key instrument." (2) "Qualitative research is descriptive." (3) "Qualitative researchers are concerned with process rather than simply with outcomes or products." (4) "Qualitative researchers tend to analyze their data inductively." (5) "'Meaning' is of essential concern to the qualitative approach." This study exhibited each of these features.

Natural Setting as Source of Data, Researcher as Instrument

My intention was to learn how programs operated when no researcher was around—not to create some kind of intervention by my presence. I wanted to understand how parents of children with disabilities thought about inclusion, not as an abstract principle but within very specific contexts.

In pursuing these intentions, I came to know 19 Wabash youth with special needs and their families over the course of the study. Among these were three pairs of siblings, each of whom had special needs. At the lower end of the age spectrum were three seven-year-olds (Ariana, Brett, and Carlton); at the opposite end were one 15-year-old (Artie) and two 16-year-olds (Gordon and Sean). The most common disability labels reported to me were five children diagnosed with cerebral palsy, three with attention-deficit hyperactivity disorder (ADHD), and three with learning disabilities. The group included four who used wheelchairs: Ariana, who had Guillain-Barré syndrome; LaToya (age 9) and Skipper (age 10), who each had multiple disabilities; and Gordon, who had cerebral palsy. LaToya was the only one who used an augmentative communication device, although nine-year-old Erica's mother had discussed this with the school district as an option.

The activities I chose to explore in depth were those that involved, on a consistent basis, one or more children that I knew had special needs. (All observations were conducted with informed consent of families and program operators. No family or program leader declined a request for an interview or an observation during the entire year of the study.) Four different kinds of activities became the subject of sustained, in-depth examination, and each is the subject of a chapter: the baseball teams associated with the Wabash Park and Recreation Department (WPRD); the Youth Recreation Center (YRC), a drop-in facility operated by the WPRD; the Girl Scouts; and the Karate Studio. Other activities in Wabash I observed, and whose leaders I spent time getting to know, were the Boy Scouts, the 4-H clubs, and a program called "Fun Days," offered to youth in two high-poverty neighborhoods by a social service agency.

Before or after the activities, I conducted formal interviews with the people in charge, in addition to informal conversations that took place while the activities were underway. Leaders usually chose to meet me in a work-place or in the spaces where the youth programs took place, whereas most parents invited me to their homes for interviews.

How I Presented Myself to Children

Fine and Sandstrom (1988, 18–21) discuss three approaches to conducting observations among children, which they call "explicit cover," "shallow cover," and "deep cover." In the first of these modes, the observer provides a "complete and detailed explanation"; in the second, it is acknowledged that research is underway, but the researcher is "vague or less than completely candid." In deep cover, the researcher does not even reveal to participants that he or she is engaged in a study.

I opted for the middle approach—shallow cover—with the children I was observing. I let them know that I was doing research, but did not wish to spell out the focus of my inquiry, because it would have unnecessarily drawn other children's attention to their peers who had special needs. I cautioned program leaders before I arrived not to tell children (including their own) that I was targeting any children in particular, but just that I was trying to get to know about the activity or organization.

When I had the opportunity to introduce myself to a group, or when individual children asked me what I was doing, I told them I was from Brewster, from the state university, and that I had picked Wabash as a community to study "what kinds of organized activities kids your age are involved in when you're not in school." This explanation made sense to them, and it was consistent with what they saw. (For instance, a few of them saw me at more than one activity.)

When I could, I took on a role comparable to the other adults in the settings; for instance, helping children in a Brownie troop with an arts and crafts project or helping to keep an eye on the kids playing basketball at the YRC. Once, a 4-H leader had to leave for a few minutes, and I agreed to keep the discussion going until she returned. I volunteered to help out as an assistant coach for a tee-ball team, and the other two coaches obliged, even giving me a highly prized T-shirt.

Description

"The data collected are in the form of words . . . rather than numbers" (Bogdan and Biklen 1992, 30). I conducted at least one formal interview with a parent (or two parents) of each of the 19 children and also with four of the youth, three of their siblings, and two of their typically developing peers. I interviewed 20 leaders of youth or recreation programs individually or in pairs, in addition to convening two small group discussions (with Girl Scout leaders and with the staff of the Boys and Girls Club of Brewster).

The findings are presented as a narrative. Direct quotations from the interviews and from my field notes bring readers vicariously into the scenes that I observed. My goal was to pay close enough attention, and record situations in enough detail, to give readers the sense of having spent time in the case study community themselves.

Numerical (as distinct from statistical) data can sometimes be useful in refining a description, and qualitative researchers are not averse to using them to enhance the descriptive power of words (Johnson and Johnson 1990). It is useful to know that Wabash was a community of roughly 14,000 people, as I have indicated, and not 1,400 or 140,000. It is informative to note that there were 19 children with special needs whom I came to know over the course of this case study and that their ages ranged, as indicated above, from 7 to 16 years.

Process Rather Than Outcomes

One could invent a variety of outcome measures related to inclusive practices in recreational settings if one were launching a different kind of inquiry. Did Boy Scouts with special needs earn a comparable number of merit badges during a week at camp compared with other boys without special needs? Did a Girl Scout with a disability get selected as frequently as her peers to carry the flag as part of the color guard? Did a coach devote equal attention to working with a child with a sensory impairment as to his teammates?

These were not the kinds of questions that animated this inquiry. I was not interested in giving a "thumbs up" or "thumbs down" to any individual program leader or organization, in accordance with any given view of what might be considered optimal inclusive practices. Rather, I was seeking understanding of the evolution of individual and organizational perspectives. I was seeking to learn how leaders, parents, and youth thought about issues, what they paid attention to, what decisions they made. I was looking for signals from either individuals or organizations that they were cognizant of the presence of youth with special needs and looking to see how their thoughts or actions reflected that recognition.

Inductive Interpretation

I did not begin with hypotheses that I was hoping to disprove or verify but with some questions and issues derived from my own experience and from the literature I had reviewed. Working inductively means sometimes altering the procedures of the inquiry on the basis of evidence one has gathered, rather than collecting data strictly in accordance with research procedures established from the outset. Illustrative of this is that I decided to gather data outside of the case study community in two instances. The family of Artie, a 15-year-old with Down Syndrome, chose to send him to a summer program in Brewster. David, a 12-year-old with ADHD, dropped out of the Boy Scout troop he attended in Wabash and rejoined a troop in a smaller nearby town where he used to live. I decided in both cases to investigate what kinds of experiences they were having in these other programs and why each family (or David himself) had made this choice. In a community where there was not a great deal of overt discussion and opinion expressed about the reasons for using or not using recreational programs, the act of getting in a car and driving to another town was a powerful statement. It impelled me to climb behind the wheel of my own car, notepad in my back pocket, and head off in the same direction.

My overall interpretive stance drew heavily from Stake (1978, 1994, 1995). Stake (1995, 74) contrasts "categorical aggregation" and "direct interpretation." To aggregate data is deliberately to lose the particularity of specific cases in favor of thematic but thinner data in order to put things in categories and draw conclusions. I had to do some aggregation in order to make sense of the enormous quantities of notes from field observations and interviews that I compiled. An example will be found in the next chapter, when I describe the economic conditions of the families with whom I met. How many of them lived in subsidized housing or lacked telephones? How many of them needed scholarship help to send their children to summer camps? How well off were these parents, on the whole? Aggregating from field notes and interviews allowed me to answer these questions and thereby help to set the stage for readers.

However, the trustworthiness of my conclusions rests ultimately not on this kind of aggregation but on direct interpretation. From among the data I gathered, I have elected to narrate in vivid detail a small number of episodes and exchanges. I do not claim that these activities or dialogues are representative of those that occurred most frequently. Put simply, they are the ones that enabled me to draw insight from the research activities in which I engaged. After sifting and thinking over many episodes and experiences that I recorded during the case study, they are the ones whose recounting I believed would provide the greatest benefit to readers.

Search for Meaning

In addition to persons directly involved in recreational programs, I arranged to meet with two ministers, a bank president, the principal of one of the four public elementary schools, the Chief of Police, the leader of a parents' association for families of children with disabilities, and the founder of a local philanthropy for low-income children. They filled in gaps in my knowledge and provided some historical background. During the writing process, I tested out my interpretations and conclusions on some of them. Soliciting their perspectives helped me to make sure that I looked at Wabash with a wider angle lens than was possible by only talking with those directly involved as consumers or operators of programs for youth.

As for those whose experiences were most central to my research, I went out of my way to ensure that their perspectives—not my own subjectivities—would shape my understandings. I tried to take the aura of mystery out of the research process, through the words I used and the ways I presented myself.

"The meaning sought in inquiry is understood only through dialogue and negotiation between the researcher and the researched. Further, researchers have the responsibility to be sensitive to the inequities of power that exist between them and those with whom they are working, for example, between university scholar and school district practitioner, or between adult and child" (Walsh, Tobin, and Graue 1993, 464).

I introduced myself to families and program leaders in Wabash just as I have to readers of this book: not as disinterested, unbiased observer but as one who was interested and biased. I confessed to being a partisan of inclusion, someone whose sister had Down Syndrome and who believed that children with disabilities were entitled to participate in their community's activities. I also explained that I was doing graduate work in education at the state university in Brewster. In that context, I hadn't come to Wabash to promote my beliefs about inclusion. I wanted to understand what kinds of problems were presented when children and youth with special needs attempted to participate in local activities, and how parents and practitioners went about addressing them. As much as was practical, I made the questions I was contemplating known to the adults in the settings I was studying. I was constantly on the lookout to understand what questions or issues they found salient.

As I completed portions of the writing, I invited adult respondents, whose words, activities, or experiences I relied on, to provide feedback as to whether their thoughts had been accurately heard, recorded, and reflected in the final product. This totaled 24 study participants (or *respondents*, as they are generally called in qualitative research). They had an opportunity to review drafts of chapters or of chapter excerpts. When children played a central role in what I wrote, it was their parents whom I invited to review and comment. Seeking this kind of feedback from participants in a qualitative study is commonly referred to as *member checking* (Lincoln and Guba 1985, 314).

Along with a section of the draft, I distributed to each respondent a one-page memorandum, in which I stated that I would pay close attention to any suggestions or corrections they made but could not "promise to make every change that you may suggest." I asked them to call to my attention any factual errors and to let me know if I had accurately presented their point of view or opinions. The memorandum continued: "Look carefully at any place where I quote you. Please feel free to write in changes if you think it does not sound like the words you would have used. Please let me know if reading this draft has sparked additional thoughts that you would like to share with me."

In each case, I telephoned, voiced the above suggestions, and explained that I was going to drop off the draft manuscript to them. I encouraged them to telephone me or write down comments, whichever was more comfortable for them. With each draft section, I dropped off an envelope addressed to me, with the correct amount of postage already affixed.

Stake has frequently used this form of member checking with those in the settings he studies. (He calls them actors.)

In long use of member checking, I typically get little back from the actor—not very satisfying but entirely necessary. I often do not have all my facts straight and I need help . . . The most frequent response of the actors to whom I sent drafts is not to acknowledge that I have sent anything . . . But sometimes I get a thorough reading, a mutually respectful argument, and suggestions for improvement. I think I can say that all my reports have been improved by member checking. (Stake 1995, 116)

I was more fortunate; I got back nearly all of them. However, the substantive results were similar to those described by Stake: a few factual corrections, a few thoughtful comments. Most found the drafts acceptable as written and returned them without any comments. A few were enthusiastic about the accuracy with which I had captured their perspectives. Nobody asked me to alter any of their direct quotations. No one quarreled with descriptions of specific episodes or with my interpretations.

It is important for readers to know of the strategies I used to gain feedback from those in the case study community and confirm that in their view, I had captured their words and experiences honestly and accurately. Still, I do not attribute the meaning I have drawn from this study, or the conclusions I have reached, to anyone but myself.

"No other issue so clearly distinguishes interpretive researchers from others than their confidence in the worth of case studies. . . . Interpretive researchers find the well done case study both interesting and persuasive," stated Walsh and his coauthors (1993, 468). In the next chapter, readers will travel into the heart of the case study community. I am confident they will find it an interesting place.

3

Entering Wabash

The town of Wabash had a population of approximately 14,000 at the time of this study. It was one of the larger towns in a county that occupied 1,000 square miles, most of which was farm land. The annual guide produced by the weekly newspaper listed 20 local churches, 16 fast-food eateries, 13 other restaurants, and 9 taverns. Wabash functioned as a small commercial hub for the trade and transport of farm products, in addition to being the location of a sizable number of manufacturing plants for a town of its size. At the McDonald's and some of the other eateries, one found small clusters of farmers and retired farmers gathered for friendly conversation during the breakfast hours. It was not unusual for professionals to have farm backgrounds: The elementary school principal I interviewed told me she used to supervise "50,000 laying hens" on a chicken farm before she took on responsibility for a different kind of flock.

The four chapters that follow this one will depict the current state of inclusive practice, as I encountered it, within four specific programs or organizations in Wabash: two operated by the town, one an affiliate of a national nonprofit organization, and the fourth, a small, independent, privately owned business. The remainder of this chapter will provide readers with some general background about the community so that they will be able to more fully appreciate and make sense of the depictions that follow.

HISTORY OF THE TOWN'S DEVELOPMENT

Three historical developments shaped the town's economy and demographics: the railroads, the expansion of the military, and the contraction of the military. The area that would later be incorporated as the town of Wabash became in the 1850s an important stop on what was then the longest railroad in existence—the 700 miles of the Illinois Central. Within just a few years of the completion of that colossal project, the farmland in the area more than quadrupled in price, and the town was incorporated and began to take shape.

Vital as the rail link was, however, the population of the town had grown to only 1,300 by 1917. That is when the federal government recognized that the corn fields of Wabash would make an ideal site for construction of runways for the taking off and landing of airplanes. Air flight had been achieved for the first time in 1903; there was no U.S. Air Force yet. Betting on the future of air power, decisions made in Washington, D.C., with the enthusiastic backing of business leaders and public officials from Wabash, transformed the landscape and the economic activity of this farming area into an important link in the rapidly expanding airborne capabilities of the American military.

Wabash grew incrementally over the next two decades, thanks to a single Air Force–related employer and then became a boom town during the World War II years. There were at least 13,000 jobs associated with the defense industry in 1940, and much of the rest of the town's economy was geared to servicing that huge complement of men and women. From the 1950s through the 1980s, thanks to the continued presence of the town's major employer, the population of the town rose to nearly 30,000.

In the 1990s, Wabash suffered the fate of dozens of cities and towns across the country that either lost military bases or saw their major employers lose contracts for the manufacture of defense and aerospace products. The USSR, whether as a real threat to U.S. security or as a bogeyman to justify military-related spending, ceased to exist. The enormous proportion of the federal budget devoted to defense for much of the post–World War II era declined. The major employer of Wabash (and the second largest employer in the county, after the state university) closed its doors over a period of several years and sold off its property. As a direct result of that, the town's population shrunk to its current level—about twice what it was before its World War II boom, but only 50 to 60 percent of what it was in the 1980s.[1]

Recovering from Loss of Jobs

At the time this study took place, the town's local government and schools, as well as many of its businesses, civic institutions, and families, were still completing a transition from the defense-related economy of previous decades to the current mixed economy. The town's three largest employers now were manufacturers of automotive plastics, wood window frames, and bicycle and motorcycle accessories. Together, these three companies employed more than 2,500 people. The unemployment rate was 3.8 percent, low for the nation as a whole but higher than the county average of only 3 percent.

The police chief, who joined the department 30 years earlier, said that, from the point of view of law enforcement, there was a definite change in population. "We were always a blue collar town, even a white collar town." Now, he said, there was a lower income level, more single-parent families, more people just scraping by, working at unskilled factory jobs, presenting different kinds of problems.

A principal of one of the elementary schools put it more dramatically. "I sometimes go to seminars on change now, and you have to laugh! What don't we know about change? We lost half our faculty, our average income went down maybe, what—20 percent? It's like the town moved, but we stayed." She mentioned that one of the schools now had about 65 percent of its students eligible for free or subsidized lunches (a standard set by the U.S. Department of Agriculture, based on federal poverty guidelines). "That was unheard of! It never would have been more than 20 to 30 percent," before the town lost its major employer. She also emphasized that there were now more obvious socioeconomic divisions among the kids coming to school. "There are the haves and the have-nots. The haves are getting picked up by a parent and going off to ballet and horseback riding. The have-nots are the ones I end up dealing with, taking them home because no one has come for them, or helping them get a bookbag or something."

The comments made by leaders of 4-H clubs, Boy Scouts, and Girl Scouts were consistent with this picture of the economic conditions of Wabash. At least one leader from each of these organizations told me that the purchase of uniforms and other items that might have been taken for granted in a more affluent community were beyond the means of a majority of the children they worked with in Wabash.[2]

Statistics from the school district report cards (required of every school district in the state) bore out the current high levels of poverty in Wabash. Using a definition adopted by the state education department for purposes of uniform reporting, the percentage of students from low-income families attending public schools in the state as a whole was 34.9 percent. A smaller town near Wabash had 11.4 percent, Jefferson City had 8.4 percent, and Brewster had 27.7 percent. In Wabash, according to the 1995 report card their officials filed, fully 48 percent of the public school students, grades K through eight, were from low-income families.

FEATURES OF COMMUNITY LIFE

Like other towns in the region, the landscape underneath and surrounding Wabash was infallibly flat and mostly bereft of trees. (These characteristics had once been strong selling points for the construction of runways.) Driving beyond the town limits in any of the four directions, one passed large tracts of farmland. The other towns one passed within a 40-mile radius in any direction were smaller than Wabash, except for Brewster, 15 miles to the south.

Brewster numbered around 100,000 people and was the seat of a state land-grant university, as well as a community college that offered classes in Wabash. For their health care, residents of Wabash patronized the two hospitals and associated medical clinics and offices in Brewster. The school department of Wabash sought new hires from the state university's teacher training programs. To judge by the quantity of advertising that Brewster's retail stores stuffed into the Wabash newspaper (and the limited number of functioning stores in Wabash), the residents of this community made frequent shopping trips to Brewster.

The two communities were connected by an older four-lane state road that ran straight north from Brewster, with barely a single curve or swerve along the route, and became the central business artery of Wabash. There was also an interstate highway running on the west side of both municipalities, with a Wabash exit that let drivers off about a mile and a half from the center of town. Either route took about 20 minutes. A half dozen of the fast-food outlets mentioned above, as well as one of the elementary schools, were located on the road running between the town center and the interstate.

The commercial center of Wabash was originally built around the train station. An Amtrak station still occupied the same location as the 1856 train station, and there was a downtown in the few blocks around it. It housed (among others) one auto dealership, two haircutters, two gift shops, one realtor, an auto parts store, a liquor store, a florist, and a furniture store. Like many downtown areas, it did not bustle with economic vitality. The storefronts that were open were well-tended, and parking was free. But some shops were empty, and none ever seemed to be bursting with patrons. The brick police and fire stations, built in the 1980s, were the newest structures. Aside from two bars, there was no place to eat in the downtown area.

Mobile Home Parks Adjacent to Private Homes

The residential neighborhoods close to downtown were older, quite modest, and with minimal yard space. Some of the private homes were doubles. To the east, leaving town, before the terrain turned into farm country, were a few of the more prosperous businesses, including a major discount store and a sports bar. Farther out in that direction were some manufacturing plants. There was also in that same area a small mall that had been closed for several years.

Working back into town from the east, one arrived at the community's sole operating mall, anchored by the town's two grocery stores and a branch of the state motor vehicle department. It was modestly busy at most times. Much of the poverty, including mobile home parks and public housing, was concentrated in areas to the north and south of this mall.

There were no rigid demarcations between neighborhoods of lower income and higher income residents. New and comparatively expensive homes were under construction west of downtown, just a few hundred feet from a crowded lot that housed 14 mobile homes. One of the more impressive houses I visited, located on a small farm property and filled with antiques and beautifully refinished woodwork (the owner was a high school vocational teacher and 4-H leader), was just a quarter of a mile down the road from another mobile home park.

Public Spaces

Distributed fairly evenly throughout the community were parks and playgrounds, many with recently acquired equipment. When I asked one of the ministers I interviewed what he liked about Wabash (he had come to his congregation from out of state three years earlier), he mentioned the number of parks and the unusually high number of children as factors that attracted him.

The community's largest outdoor sports complex (baseball diamonds, basketball courts, playground with lighting for evening usage) was located adjacent to its largest public housing development. There were also a few small lakes—one located in the town's largest green space, inherited from the town's one-time major employer, at the southern end of the community, and two others abutting some of the more affluent residential streets at the western edge of the residential neighborhoods.

Some of the publicly operated recreational facilities were clustered together close to the center of town. The municipal swimming pool sat next to a large public park with four baseball diamonds where most of the baseball leagues met to play. These spaces abutted the high school on one side; private homes were just across the street. Other recreational facilities, including the Youth Recreation Center (the focus of a later chapter), had been acquired from the town's former major employer and were therefore located away from the residential neighborhoods in the southern part of the community.

On the whole, a good portion of the housing around the town (other than the obvious pockets of poverty) looked attractive if unpretentious, while the retail business sector looked frayed around the edges. A bank president I spoke with expressed great confidence in the housing stock of the community and cautious optimism about the future of the town's business sector. It looked like what it was: a town that may have seen better times and had no surplus of people with extra spending money, but where most neighborhoods were very livable and where the public spaces and buildings seemed more abundant and better outfitted than you might expect in a community of this size.

TOLERANCE OF DIFFERENCES—IN ETHNIC BACKGROUNDS AND ABILITIES

An interesting assertion was made to me by several parents and some of the community leaders I interviewed. They stated that there was an enduring benefit from the three generations the town had been associated with its major military-related employer. This history, they explained, had left the residents of Wabash more comfortable with racial and ethnic diversity than were the residents of other comparably sized midwestern towns. This in turn, they perceived, created a receptive climate for people with disabilities or divergent developmental needs.

Outside of Brewster (which had 37 percent nonwhite students), Wabash was the only town in the area with a racially diverse population. According to the 1995 school report card filed by the Wabash public schools, 24 percent of the students, grades kindergarten through eight, were African American (and another 3 percent Hispanic). The smaller town nearby, by contrast, reported it had only one nonwhite student out of an elementary enrollment of 329. Jefferson City, a larger town, reported 1.5 percent nonwhite enrollment.

Not only did Wabash have a considerably more racially diverse population than any other town in the area outside of Brewster, but it seemed a disproportionate number of its residents had lived in other states and even (by way of military service) in other countries. Wabash residents I met in the course of this study had lived in Okinawa, Hawaii, Alaska, Colorado, New Mexico, Arizona, Texas, Tennessee, North Carolina, and New York, as well as other midwestern states. Many had spent part or all of their childhoods in or near Wabash, then left and later returned.

Among the 19 kids with disabilities I came to know in this study were two (Carlton and LaToya) who were African American but whose foster or adoptive parents were white (i.e., of European descent). This was also the case with Lindy, whom I do not count among the 19 because she died before I undertook the research. The comments I heard from these parents left me with the impression that they felt it was somewhat easier to sustain a racially mixed family here in Wabash than in many other small-sized cities and towns.

"We Treated Him Just Like Anyone Else"

The small-town, farm-belt character of the community, with its traditional connotations of self-reliance and voluntary mutual aid, seemed to be a plus at times for children with special needs and their families. Illustrations of the good-will of the community toward those in need arose during the study. A full weekend of fund-raising activities was organized to help one long-time town resident who had been diagnosed with cancer. These efforts produced $10,000 to help this father of young children to defray his medical bills.

A local toddler was diagnosed with a hereditary disorder that would require a liver transplant, costing as much as $100,000. Stores all over town put out collection boxes. There were also roast beef dinners, country and western music concerts, raffles, and other fund-raising events. The money was collected, a donor was found, and the transplant was pronounced a success one year later.

Since Harold's birth with Down Syndrome almost two years earlier, his mother, Corinne, had been welcomed into many Wabash churches and other organizations as a speaker on the rights and needs of children with developmental differences. In contrast, when she first learned of her baby's disability, she did not get a positive response from her doctor, located in Brewster. "I found out he would be born with Down Syndrome while I was still pregnant. My obstetrician told me the baby would never reach beyond the level of a two-year-old. She strongly suggested that I abort; in fact, she didn't even act as though there was room for any other decision." It was Corinne's opinion that if she and her husband had remained in Brewster (where she had lived until a few years earlier), there never would have been the same level of community-wide recognition and acceptance that greeted them in Wabash.

Two different informants told me on separate occasions about a man with a physical disability that they had known since he was a schoolboy. One of my informants was older and had coached him; the other grew up and went to the local Catholic school with him. They said that his hands were congenitally malformed, with nubs instead of fingers. Both informants stressed that this man excelled as an athlete in spite of his disability, and each recalled his ability to shoot the basketball from the outside perimeter with great accuracy. (The one who was his contemporary added, smiling, "If you could have seen him drive, swig a beer, and smoke a cigarette. . . . ") Also, both men emphasized that he was treated just like anyone else, neither expecting nor receiving any special favors. They seemed to have drawn the lesson that this was the way to respect the dignity of a person with a disability.

Former Star Athlete Becomes Wheelchair User

I was told that the former basketball player still lived in Wabash and worked as a supervisor at one of the local manufacturing plants, but I never met him. I did meet Bill, whose experience with disability was more recent and more dramatic. Bill had been a high school athlete, well-known throughout the community for his cross-country running. In the fall of his senior year, he and a female companion had left the homecoming festivities to tow one of the floats that had been exhibited in the parade back to a farm, out in the countryside. As they pulled out onto a rural road, they became victims of a frequent cause of accidents at that time of year: obstructed visibility at an intersection, due to the height of the fully grown corn. His companion emerged, after a scare, without any serious injuries. But Bill became the first student at the high school to use a wheelchair.

One of the ministers I interviewed told me that Bill was "almost an ambassador for people with disabilities, whether he wants to be or not."

There was no doubt the community had been receptive to Bill. "It's at least partly because it's Bill—and he was so well-known!" Bill seemed to share that sentiment, saying, when I asked how people had responded to him as a person using a wheelchair, "Everybody around here knows me." He didn't feel anybody had shown him any disrespect. He shared a home in a nearby small town with one of his brothers and was proud of being able to get around town on his own, packing his wheelchair in and out of his sport utility vehicle.

No Utopia

The degree of racial diversity and the community's apparent sympathy toward children and adults with disabilities or medical problems was worthy of acknowledgment. But Wabash was no utopia: Neither racial tolerance nor positive attitudes toward those with disabilities could be assumed at all times. We have already described in Chapter 1 the encounter Lindy's parents had in the bleachers during a softball game with one apparently prejudiced grandparent. While I was completing this case study, an item appeared in the newspaper about a white, male, 17-year-old Wabash high school student who pleaded guilty in district court to committing a hate crime, which involved verbal and physical harassment of a female African American student.

The same minister who described Bill as a kind of ambassador also told me that for at least 10 years, the local ministerial association had identified voluntary racial segregation as an unfortunate but persistent reality, nagging at their conception of the community as one where people appreciated and respected differences. "Why, in a town of this size, do there have to be white churches and black churches?"

Another respondent told me of a problem she had some years earlier when some of the congregants, and even a clergyman at her church, made it clear that her son, who made noises at unpredictable times, was not welcome during Sunday services. This was very painful for her; unless she brought her son with her, she could not attend services herself. Fortunately for her, an invitation to her and her son to attend services at a different church was extended right away, and the congregants and minister there made them feel welcome.

HOW DID I DEFINE "CHILDREN WITH SPECIAL NEEDS"?

I did not rely on any formal coding or definitional scheme to exclude or include any particular child as a focus of this inquiry. The children on

whom I focused this inquiry were all brought to my attention by someone—a parent, a program leader, or both—who considered them to
have a disability or special needs. Because my interest was in knowing
how respondents looked on the inclusion in youth programs of children they perceived as having special needs, I did not want to define for
them which children should or should not be considered members of
that category.

Schools, Families, Youth Leaders—A Variety of Perspectives on "Special Needs"

Not all the children whom I viewed in this study as having disabilities
or special needs were enrolled in special education. Ariana had become
ill and stopped walking soon after she first learned to do so, around age
one, and had been using braces and a wheelchair ever since. She had
been classified as a special education student from age three through
kindergarten, but when I met her, she was not receiving special education services. Instead, she had a "504 plan" at school; that is, a plan (required under Section 504 of the Rehabilitation Act of 1973 because the
school district was a recipient of federal dollars) recognizing that, due
to her disability, she was entitled to extra help with her mobility around
the school—but not with her educational program.

David was in special education. He had been diagnosed as having
learning disabilities and ADHD, for the latter of which he was on medication. But his mother asserted that the diagnosis of ADHD was based
on a teacher's observations and not on a true medical examination. She
referred to David (in front of him) as an "ordinary, ornery" kid, and she
was very critical not only of doctors but of most of the school personnel
as well. She did not view him as having either a disability or special
needs. The scout leader who brought him to my attention, in contrast,
viewed David as exemplary of the challenging behaviors associated with
the label of ADHD. He most likely didn't know that David also had a
label of learning disabilities when he went to school.

Trying to impose a predetermined definition of special needs (of my
own making or one drawn from the literature) would in all likelihood
have been a futile exercise. Consider the experience that Bogdan and
Kugelmass (1984, 174) had with definitional problems in a study they
conducted. "As we entered the schools to start our observations, a clear
concept of disability, mainstreaming and special education turned more
and more into a mirage." They go on to explain:

The ways children are perceived, including whether they are thought of as handicapped . . . vary from school district to school district, from school to school, and from place to place within a given school. In addition, who was considered handicapped and what specific type of handicapping conditions a student has, varies from time to time. . . . The assignment of a label of exceptionality has as much to do with the situation a child finds him/herself in as it does with the child him/herself. (175–176)

Because my inquiry concerned the experiences of youth in more informal and recreational settings, not in schools, it made the definitional issues even more murky than the study described in the passage above. School districts follow federal and state laws in diagnosing and categorizing students for educational purposes (even though they don't all interpret the laws in the same ways). But the recreation and youth programs in Wabash (as in most other places) did not ask families, in connection with the enrollment of their children, to identify children's disabilities or their placement in special education.

Restrictions on Sharing Information

A school principal told me it would be a violation of confidentiality for her to inform the director of the Youth Recreation Center (YRC) whether a child they both worked with was in special education. Greg, the director of the YRC, similarly acknowledged that he usually did not have this information. What he did know was which children presented the most troubling behaviors at the YRC. When I asked him about "kids with special needs or disabilities" who spent time at the center, those are the ones that came to mind.

Greg told me that Ginny Riley was one of his most challenging participants, due to her occasional outbursts of aggression and defiance. I sought out and interviewed her mother, and for the purposes of this book, I considered Ginny as a "child with special needs." Yet I learned from her mother that she had never been in special education and had never been otherwise labeled as having any kind of disability. (She had, however, repeated a grade.)

Rather than simply describing a child using a label that was reported to me as if it were an immutable artifact, I explain throughout this book (as in this discussion) whether it was a label assigned to the child in school, a doctor's diagnosis as reported by a parent, an informed guess on the part of a youth program leader, or originated in some other fashion. In providing this kind of contextual background, I hope to assist readers in developing accurate perceptions of the youth whom I describe and to help them recognize the complexity of the problem of defining who does and who does not have special needs or disabilities.

GETTING TO KNOW THE FAMILIES OF CHILDREN WITH DISABILITIES

The parents of the 19 Wabash children with special needs[3] I came to know were mostly wage earners with modest incomes. From my observations, they ranged from just getting by (or not quite getting by) to reasonably secure, but I saw and heard no evidence of abundance or luxury. One family added what appeared to be costly renovations to an already spacious home during the study; but that family had eight children (including some foster children). The majority of the others owned their own homes, all of modest size, with small yards, and neatly but unpretentiously furnished. The vans that three families needed to transport children who used wheelchairs were among the more lavish possessions I noted. (The family of the fourth child who used a wheelchair could not afford a van.) One family gave me as their reason for relocating from Brewster the fact that they could afford their own home in Wabash. Yet Brewster itself had been listed in a national survey as a city with some of the most affordable housing stock in the country.

Two families of children with special needs—one a single mom, the other a couple with two children with special needs—did not have telephones. Both lived in subsidized housing. One of these parents commented that "if it wasn't for the free store, there'd be no way to get clothes at all." (The reference was to a church-sponsored store.) They had recently bought a used car, but it was leaking oil, and they could not afford to get it fixed.

Another married couple and their son lived in a mobile-home park, of which there were several in Wabash. This family had moved several times in recent years. I did not learn the nature of the husband's employment (the wife was not employed), but trappings of material success were not in evidence, either inside or outside their home. As I got into my car after an interview there, another motorist beeped and asked which unit was the source for buying drugs. She had spied a well-groomed, unfamiliar, middle-aged man with a new car and apparently ruled out any other explanation for my presence in that location.

Two families among those I studied sent their children to a week of special summer camp. In both cases, this rested on the availability of scholarship assistance. A third mentioned that a camp they were interested in for their son was not affordable.

Here are some of the jobs held by the mothers (and one grandmother) of the youth with special needs: three registered nurses, three production workers in factories, part-time worker at a motel, manager of a deli at the main supermarket in town, housecleaner for a sorority in Brewster, social service project supervisor.

Here are some of the jobs held by the fathers: water department technician for the town of Wabash, superintendent at a factory, maintenance man for an apartment complex, photocopy machine repairman, laborer, broadcast engineer for a television station in Brewster, beer distributor, minister.

Encounters with Hospitals and the Health Care System

Many of these families had spent a great portion of their energy and time (and financial resources, too) facing, addressing, and advocating for diagnoses, treatment, and therapies for their children. Three of them had come face-to-face with the possible or actual deaths of their children. Lindy, whose story we have recounted, died at age 12, three months before the study began. Rosemary's son Peter, about whom we shall learn more later on, also died at age 12, two years prior to the study. A third family had faced the possible loss of their typically developing son Skipper, at age seven (three years prior to the case study), when he became asphyxiated during a playground accident. After he recovered, but with multiple and severe disabilities, the family moved to Wabash in order to be near the medical facilities of Brewster. They came from a rural area, three hours away.

Most of the time, parents of youth with special needs were not dealing with life and death. But serious encounters with hospitals and the medical system—encounters that left several of them frustrated or even embittered—made up an important part of the narratives of their lives.

Ariana's parents went through years of anxiety before they got either an appropriate diagnosis for their daughter[4] or any effective response to her condition. When she became ill with flu-like symptoms at the age of 10 months, they brought her in, several weeks in a row, and reported their growing alarm at her seeming regression in development. Instead of following her situation more closely, the doctor in their managed-care plan criticized them for being overprotective. The physician's explanation for her regressions was that Ariana was in a lazy stage; he advised the parents to calm down. Only after they had relocated to Wabash from another part of the state and a more empathetic doctor in a different medical group referred them to a neurologist did anyone pay heed to their observations. The real breakthrough didn't come until she was three years old, when they took her to the Shriners' hospital in a neighboring state. That's when Ariana was finally diagnosed with Guillain-Barré syndrome. When I met her, she used a wheelchair during her recreational hours (or sat on the floor) and practiced at school on increasing the use of braces.

Tara had the experience of being told by a physician that her son Brett, who was a late developing baby, had cerebral palsy and that he would use a wheelchair for the rest of his life. In fact, he never had to use a wheelchair at all; he learned to walk unassisted but with an awkward gait. When I interviewed Tara and her husband, they were facing an imminent decision about whether Brett should undergo another round of surgery.

The following is from my interview notes: "Adam has heard Tara scheduling talks with doctors about his hips. He has said, 'I'm not having another surgery!' She has said, 'but if it will help you to walk straighter and maybe even help you run?' 'But you're not the one who had to go through it! I don't want to go through the pain.' "

Jennifer's parents had no trouble getting the correct diagnosis for her; that is, that she was deaf. But that was because they made arrangements on their own to have her hearing tested when she was only two days old. They did not want to repeat the unhappy experience they had with her older brother: They told me it took doctors six months to diagnose Colin's deafness. In later years, they faced another kind of anxiety but this time in part self-imposed. They decided to have both children undergo surgery for cochlear implants (to give them some auditory capacity), during a time when it was still regarded as experimental (and frowned on by many who regarded themselves as members of a deaf community).

Erica had cerebral palsy, but like so many other children with disabilities, her primary diagnosis was not the only source of her health problems. On her first birthday, her mom and dad had to bring her to the hospital for heart surgery. Erica's mom later went back to school and became a nurse because, "I wanted to know what they were saying about my child."

Gordon was a 16-year-old high school student whose encounters with the medical system were benign but nonetheless pivotal among his childhood memories. He could tell me his exact age (not just the year but the month) on the occasions of his three major surgeries. He could also explain in each instance what muscles or ligaments were operated on, what the purpose of each operation was, and exactly how much school he missed in each situation.

Carlton missed the team photo for his tee-ball team becaused he was rushed to the hospital in Brewster on account of a seizure. The first time I visited LaToya's mom, she had kept LaToya home from school and periodically excused herself to check on how she was responding to a new formula that she was trying in her feeding tube. The medical and developmental needs of this group of children were seldom far from their parents' minds.

Identifying and Coming to Terms with Special Needs: A Process, Not an Event

Only a few of the children in the case-study community were identified at birth as having special needs. Four started out developing normally but acquired disabilities through illness or injury. Ariana became ill at age 10 months with Guillain-Barré syndrome. Cliff lost 60 percent of his hearing at age two as a result of a high fever. Rosemary's son Peter had a near-SIDS (Sudden Infant Death Syndrome) experience at age four and one-half months. Skipper, as we have described, became asphyxiated at age seven in a playground accident.

Erica and Brett, each of whom had cerebral palsy, were not diagnosed until they were emerging from infancy and showing signs of developmental delay. Others who were eventually diagnosed with ADHD or learning disabilities did not show evidence of these problems until they reached school age. Five of the 19 had been adopted (Lindy, La-Toya, Henry, Artie) or in foster care (Carlton); thus, their complete histories were not known by their current families.

As these numerous examples illustrate, no matter when the parents first learned about the disability or special needs, and no matter when the children first acquired their disabilities, understanding the nature of the special needs of the children was a slow, unfolding process. Gaining knowledge about the nature of their children's individual needs took time, energy, and sometimes financial resources. Securing appropriate health care and therapies, and making major medical decisions (e.g., whether to have surgery) was a central part of several of these families' experiences. After resolving these emotionally draining considerations (or sometimes while they were still trying to resolve them), the parents faced other important questions that parents of typically developing youth also faced of which one was: Where will my child go to school?

Schooling and Special Education in Wabash

There were four elementary schools, one junior high, and one high school in Wabash. The high school served a larger geographic area and was under a separate township administration, while the elementary and junior high schools served only children from the town of Wabash itself (plus 25 special education students contracted in from smaller towns). Total enrollment in the five schools was approximately 1,400. There was also a Catholic school that served approximately 175 students from grade one through grade eight; those children came from Wabash and surrounding towns.

Until 1994, the Wabash schools placed many of their special education students out of district. Students, ages five and up, who were classified as educable mentally handicapped (EMH) and trainable mentally handicapped (TMH) and some others, were bussed to the public schools in Brewster. Meanwhile, three-to five-year-olds with developmental delays from Wabash, as well as preschoolers eligible for a state-funded prekindergarten program for students at risk of academic failure, went to a specially designed preschool on the campus of the state university.

In 1994–95, the district began serving special education students with nearly all types of disabilities within their own buildings. In response to a written query, the assistant superintendent reported to me that only seven students from grades kindergarten through eight were placed out of district in 1995–96; these were children with hearing impairment or deafness, or vision impairment or blindness.[5]

In 1995–96, 220 Wabash children were served as special education students within the five schools, grades K to eight, or nearly 16 percent of all their pupils. This proportion was much greater than the approximately 10.6 percent of all students enrolled in school, ages 6 through 17 nationwide, or the 10.9 percent statewide who received special education services in 1995–96 (U.S. Department of Education 1997, A-37). However, this disproportion is in part due to the fact that several smaller school districts surrounding Wabash placed special education students in classes in Wabash, just as Wabash continued to place a few students in Brewster.

Of the Wabash youngsters, 65 percent were classified as having learning disabilities. This compared with 51.3 percent of the special education students, ages 6 through 17, nationwide, and to just under 51 percent who were classified as having specific learning disabilities in the state in which Wabash was located. Nationally, another 20.3 percent had speech or language impairments, and statewide, this figure was 23 percent (U.S. Department of Education 1997, A-34). According to the information they provided to me, however, the Wabash schools did not use the label of speech- or language-impaired for any of their special education students from kindergarten through junior high, even though its frequent usage by school districts across the country made that category the second most commonly used classification in special education.

The percentages in Wabash for mental retardation (combining the EMH and TMH categories) and behavior disorders[6] were 22 percent and 13 percent of the special education population, respectively, compared with 11.3 percent and 8.7 percent for the nation and 9.9 perent and 11.8 percent for the state (U.S. Department of Education 1997, A-34). In sum, the Wabash schools found a slightly higher percentage of their student body eligible for special education; used the learning disabilities, mental retardation, and behavior disorders classifications disproportionately; and did not use the speech or language impairment category at all, in comparison with the state and the nation.

Some of the children were a living testament to the evolving practices of the school district. Gordon had been bussed to Brewster for school until sixth grade, even though his only disabilities were physical. (He was the first student who entered the high school in Wabash in a wheelchair. Bill, the former cross-country runner, had also used a wheelchair, but only during his senior year after the accident that paralyzed his legs.) Several of the children I met had been part of the cohort who had been bussed to the state university preschool in their early years. Jennifer was one of the seven Wabash children whom the school district continued to transport to Brewster. There, she was included in regular middle school classes, with sign language interpreters available to accompany her and other deaf students from all over the county.

Even with their children staying mostly in Wabash for their schooling, many of these parents faced difficult educational decisions and responsibilities. LaToya used an alternative communication device (called a Liberator), with a head switch to activate it, because she had very limited dexterity in her hands. Her mom's job was to keep the teachers up-to-date on what words and phrases were programmed into the Liberator. Erica's situation was complicated by the fact that therapists and educators were unsure what type of communication (oral language or sign language) they should concentrate on teaching her. Her mom didn't want to insist the school purchase her an augmentative communication device (which was very expensive) if it wasn't needed, but she worried equally that if it really were needed, perhaps she should be a little more pushy about it.

Lucas's mom was certain that her son needed specialized instructional approaches and was not confident the Wabash schools had figured out the right ones (although she appreciated their efforts). She had taken him out of the public schools and put him in the Catholic school in Wabash for one year, because he was so far behind in reading. There, he fell even further behind. She transferred him back into public school; she was becoming desperate.

Neighborhood Schools, Separate Experiences

Lindy's mom reported that the "worst thing Lindy ever had to deal with, over the 12 years of her life, was having to have her mom or dad in school at lunch time" to give her an insulin injection, "because she knew that none of the other kids had their parents there." (They could have insisted that the school arrange for a nurse or home health aide to do it, but they did not choose to have a confrontation over it.)

Most special education students in Wabash, even though they were now attending schools in their own community, were assigned to separate classes for most of the day. (Students with learning disabilities were the major exception to this rule.) Thus, many of them faced the same experience that Lindy's mother had described—that of being looked on as noticeably different from their peers. A principal whom I interviewed said the district had been moving more children with behavior disorders into regular classrooms for an increasing amount of the time and finding most of them doing surprisingly well. Progress clearly continued, incrementally, year by year, in the direction of greater inclusion.

What remained true for many of the children was this: The assumption that they could and should participate on an equal footing with typically developing peers did not operate in their daily school routines. One of the aims of my investigation was to find out whether it operated in the recreational settings where I sought to observe them.

4

Batter Up? Fun Versus Competition in the Park and Recreation Department's Baseball Leagues

The Wabash Park and Recreation Department (WPRD), with seven full-time staff, plus part-timers and volunteers, operated a wide range of programs for all ages. It combined resources with two other public entities—the park district, a taxing body independent of the municipality, and the high school, which fell under township administration—to provide staffing and maintenance of athletic fields, playgrounds, and facilities throughout the community.

For adults, it offered aerobics, woodworking, ceramics, and many other classes, as well as seasonal sports leagues. For children, it offered instructional classes such as ballet and martial arts, sports camps, and sports leagues. During the summer, the WPRD operated a golf course and an outdoor swimming pool, where it sponsored Red Cross–approved instructional swimming, as well as novice swimming and general, family swimming. Year-round, it also invited participation in a wide variety of special events: for instance, bringing youth to the annual All Night Ski Event sponsored by the state Recreation and Park Association.

In addition, the department operated two membership-based facilities: one for adults and one for youth under age 16. In the former, there were accommodations for running, exercise equipment, weight lifting, and a gym. The latter, the Youth Recreation Center (YRC), offered drop-in recreation for youth ages 7 to 15 after school and on weekends, seven days a week, plus extended hours during summers and other times when schools were not in session.

Chapter 5 is devoted to a discussion of the YRC. This chapter concentrates on the participation of youth with special needs in sports teams sponsored by the WPRD.

HOW A SMALL-TOWN DEPARTMENT RESPONDED TO THE NEW CHALLENGES

When I informed Drew, the department's program director, of my interest in learning about the participation of youth with special needs in their activities, the first thing he mentioned was that the department had renovated some of the playgrounds in accordance with the standards of the Americans with Disabilities Act. He offered to arrange a tour, and when he drove me around, he pointed out some of the features that were added or built-in to ensure accessibility.

Drew was a trim man just entering middle age, who dressed casually and nearly always sported sneakers and a baseball cap, befitting the mix of managerial functions and blue collar work that made up his time on the job. From trying to see him many times, I learned that he did not spend large blocks of time in his office. On my first attempt to introduce myself to him in early spring, his assistant told me I could find him "hanging hoops" in the adult fitness facility. When the summer season approached, he didn't have a crew of underlings to put to work readying the municipal swimming pool: He was in and around the empty pool, cleaning it himself. His job kept him moving around, keeping tabs on the people, activities, and facilities associated with his department. He seemed to like it that way.

Legal Requirements Fulfilled—But How Much Did They Accomplish?

Proudly Drew touted to a visiting researcher that the town of Wabash, in spite of its small size, was meeting national disability standards. But he also professed, in a quiet way, to finding the logic of some of the design changes rather elusive. For instance, he pointed to a play structure at one park that was built with ramps that would allow a child in a wheelchair to make use of it. But he wasn't sure "how much good it did," since, to reach it, you had to first get across an area covered with wood chips, which would be impossible in a wheelchair.

One of the renovated playgrounds Drew showed me was located about 20 feet from the front door of the YRC, just off the driveway, where parents pulled up to drop off and pick up their children. The price tag for the colorful, state-of-the-art molded plastic climbing structures, surfaced with pebbles, was reported as $30,000, according to an article in the town's weekly newspaper. The funds came from the park district. From what I observed, it got very little use. The activities available inside the center and the open land beyond the playground seemed to be much more attractive to most children, most of the time, than the expensive, new, architecturally correct play structures.

A structural adaptation Drew pointed out to me was a hydraulic device that had been installed at the municipal swimming pool to enable a person who was nonambulatory to get in and out of the water. He described it as "kind of a large diaper" made of canvas that the person could lie back in or sit in while being hoisted down or up. He volunteered the comment that it "doesn't give a person a lot of dignity." Drew knew of only one young person in Wabash who had used the lift since it was installed several years earlier. That was Gordon, the 16-year-old I interviewed, the only student at the local high school who used a wheelchair.

I knew from speaking with Gordon that he had not been swimming for more than a year. Although he did not say explicitly that he had avoided the pool because he disliked using the hydraulic lift, he referred to it as something designed "for senior citizens." I interpreted this to mean that it made him feel passive and dependent—not something for a healthy adolescent. This was evidence in my mind that Drew's perception was on the mark about how using the lift might make someone feel.

Drew evidently subscribed to and read articles from publications related to recreation and parks. On a couple of occasions, he passed on articles to me that he thought I might find interesting. After our tour of the pool, he mentioned that he had read about a more state-of-the-art approach to swimming pool accessibility, called zero depth. Zero depth pools, he explained, had floors that lowered gradually from the edge of the pool, without any dramatic drop-offs in depth. A nonambulatory person could slide into and pull themselves out of the water in such pools much more independently.

Employment

Another issue that Drew brought up without waiting for me to ask was employment. He told me about Keith, a man in his mid-twenties with developmental disabilities who worked for the department. Keith's job was to do mopping and cleaning tasks at the YRC during the hours prior to the arrival of the rest of the staff. He had grown up in Wabash and (like all students who were labeled by the school district as mentally retarded, prior to 1995) had been bussed to school in Brewster. The young man was originally placed into this position with the support of a job coach, in connection with a project sponsored by the state. "But he's a local boy," Drew said. "We knew him; we knew he was responsible. His parents drop him off and pick him up. We told them there was no need to spend all that money, having the job coach stop by to do the job with him. He'll be fine." The support from the state program was phased out. Drew reported proudly that Keith had been given his own key to unlock the YRC.

Keith was not the only person with a disability who benefited from the employment practices of the WPRD. Another "local boy" in his twenties who worked for the department was Bill, a former athlete who had become disabled while in his senior year at Wabash High School, as described in Chapter 3. He was hired part-time to help supervise at the YRC.

During the summer, when Drew needed someone to deliver and pick up the equipment for the tee-ball games, which were held on a field in a different part of town from where the rest of the baseball and softball games were played, Drew hired Cliff, a 13-year-old boy with a hearing impairment. He wore hearing aids in both ears, which had shortened his baseball career. (He told me that wearing a batting helmet sometimes caused a whistling sound through his hearing devices.)

The part-time employment of two adults and one young adolescent with special needs had come about serendipitously but certainly demonstrated a degree of sensitivity and fairness toward persons with disabilities. The tour had shown me that physical accessibility (regarding playgrounds and the swimming pool) had also been on the minds of the department's leadership in the recent past. With regard to the issue that had brought me to Wabash, however—including children who had special needs as participants in the department's youth programs and activities—a similar level of past concern was not in evidence. A look back in history will help us to situate the Wabash experience I encountered within a broader context.

HISTORICAL PERSPECTIVE

Not unlike in school classrooms, the historical sequence in recreational settings proceeded from the total exclusion of youth (and adults) with disabilities to the proliferation of specialized, segregated programs and only recently to the emergence of what was referred to in the 1990s as inclusive programming. Summer camps for children and adolescents first appeared in the United States in 1861, but children with disabilities did not participate. When camps for children and youth with disabilities came into existence in the 1940s, they were set up exclusively for those with disabilities, often at the initiative of parents' associations (Schleien and Ray 1988). As recently as 1978, a special issue of *Therapeutic Recreation Journal* was devoted to camping, and "all of the articles referred to segregated camping programs designed for specific disability populations" (Sable 1992, 39).

The Playground Association of America (later renamed the National Recreation Association and then the National Recreation and Park Association), founded in 1906, helped to promote the idea that recreational services were for all people, including those who had physical disabilities (Schleien and Ray 1988). For the time period, this was a major advance in acknowledging the humanity of individuals whose appearance or development departed from what was viewed as the norm in American society. But the idea that activities could be made available to the people with and without disabilities at the same time and in the same place had not yet arrived and would not be widely embraced, in fact, until the very last decade of the century.

Returning War Veterans in the 1940s

The post–World War II era, when military veterans reentered society, set the stage for many of the more recent changes (Moon, Hart, Komissar, and Friedlander 1995). Unlike the majority of persons with disabilities in previous generations, these veterans were viewed sympathetically by American society, in spite of physical, cognitive, and emotional disabilities. "Before the war, individuals with disabilities were considered a burden to society. Inasmuch as disabled veterans were previously able-bodied individuals and accepted by society, they were considered normal even though they had become physically impaired" (DePauw and Gavron 1995, 36).

The National American Red Cross began offering recreational opportunities for these veterans even while the war was still ongoing. The Veterans' Administration was a pioneer in providing recreational services in the postwar years to its patients in hospitals and state institutions (Schleien and Ray 1988). Sir Ludwig Guttman, director of the Spinal Injury Center at Stoke Mandeville Hospital in Aylesbury, England, is credited with introducing competitive sports for veterans who had become disabled (DePauw and Gavron 1995, 36–42). He organized an archery competition in 1948, and wheelchair basketball was featured at the international Stoke Mandeville Games in 1952. Therapeutic horseback riding was started by doctors in the United States and other countries in the 1950s.

All these activities geared to persons with disabilities marked an important step forward in the access of these men (and some women) to a fuller, more well-rounded life experience. Nonetheless, it is important to recognize that those developing these services viewed them as a form of rehabilitation—a connotation that recreation did not have for the rest of the population. The term *therapeutic recreation* first appeared in the literature in the 1950s (DePauw and Gavron 1995) as a term of art to denote recreational programs that were specially designed for rehabilitative purposes for persons with injuries, illnesses, or disabilities.

Even while many service providers continued to view recreation for persons with special needs strictly as a way of achieving the more valued goal of rehabilitation, adults with disabilities themselves began adapting sports and recreation activities and organizing leagues and competitions. Sports enthusiasts among the population of men and women who had disabilities in the United States and Europe founded the National Wheelchair Athletic Association in 1957, the International Sports Organization for the Disabled in 1963, and the International Cerebral Palsy Society in 1968 (DePauw and Gavron 1995, 43). Their reasons were indistinguishable from those of their nondisabled contemporaries: "so that they could become fit, develop hobbies, and participate in community or team endeavors" (Moon, Hart, Komissar, and Friedlander 1995, 1). On the legislative front, the culmination of their efforts may be seen as the passage of P.L. 95–606, the Amateur Sports Act of 1978. This brought amateur athletic competition for persons with disabilities formally into the Olympic movement as of 1979. In that arena, the historic connection of the athletic endeavors of persons with disabilities to therapy was eroded, if not completely washed away.

Deinstitutionalization in the 1970s and 1980s

From 1967 to 1987, the population living in residential institutions for persons with mental retardation shrank nationwide by more than 50 percent, from almost 195,000 to fewer than 95,000 (Schleien, Tabourne, and Dart 1995, 5). Formerly housed together and provided recreational opportunities in residential institutions, or in special recreation programs sponsored by park districts, they were now dispersed into the community living independently or with their families. Park districts and other local recreation providers were increasingly in contact with persons with mental disabilities. Families were aware of their responsibility to respond to this part of the citizenry.

Progress toward inclusive practices was incremental and uneven. A survey of 552 agencies (park and recreation, public schools, and community recreation) in Minnesota in the early 1980s found that fewer than half the responding agencies brought participants with and without disabilities together for "games, entertainment, arts and crafts, and swimming." As for camping and nature activities, not even 10 percent of responding agencies at that time practiced inclusive programming (Schleien and Werder 1985, 57).

Yet during the same decade, the preferences of consumers who had disabilities were irrevocably moving in the direction of inclusion. In a survey of individuals with disabilities conducted by a county recreation department in Maryland, 90 percent of the 6,000 respondents said they would prefer to be involved in regular programs available to the public, rather than "special" recreation activities (Richardson, Wilson, Wetherald, and Peters 1987).

Some municipal recreation and park agencies began wholeheartedly to embrace inclusive programming in the 1990s. "The tide is changing! We at Chapel Hill Parks and Recreation have adopted a new philosophy" exclaimed a notice in a 1990 bulletin of the Chapel Hill, North Carolina, Parks and Recreation Department: "The Department has restructured the 'Special Populations' Recreation Specialist position into a Mainstream Coordinator position. The Mainstream Coordinator is responsible for identifying the resources that may be needed to make all our recreation programs accessible to persons with disabilities."

In a similar vein, a brochure distributed in Hazelwood, Missouri, in 1995 (Coordinator of Inclusive Recreation, n.d.), asked patrons of its Recreation Department, "Do you have a disability? Are you looking for recreation programs? A coordinator of inclusive recreation has been hired by four municipalities to help them include people of all abilities into their programs." It went on to specify that persons with disabilities could participate in any program offered by the departments of these four separate towns, and the patrons or program leaders could call on help from a newly hired staff member.

THE PRESENCE—AND ABSENCE—OF CHILDREN WITH SPECIAL NEEDS ON WPRD BASEBALL AND SOFTBALL TEAMS

Colin, who was deaf, was 17 at the time of the study. (He was the older brother of Jennifer, whose experiences in Girl Scouts are described in a later chapter.) I learned from his family that he played baseball in the WPRD leagues several years earlier, when he was between the ages of 7 and 10. The parents attributed the positive nature of the experience not to any particular values or attitudes promoted by the WPRD itself but to the sensitivity of the particular coach to whose team he had been assigned, a man they knew from church. The same gentleman coached Colin all three years, and very approvingly, Colin's dad gave him credit for teaching his son how to hit a pitched ball.

Although the experience sounded like a positive one for Colin, it had its hardships from the parents' perspective. Colin had problems with balance associated with his hearing loss, which caused him to run awkwardly. His mom and dad recalled other parents making insulting comments about his running, not knowing Colin's parents were nearby. His mom said she "told off" someone once and then started bringing a lawn chair so she wouldn't have to sit on the bleachers and risk hearing that kind of comment. Colin's dad commented that it was too bad so many parents were "out for blood" when youth sports were supposed to be for fun.

The reason Colin stopped playing baseball, however, was unrelated to any problems he or his parents encountered. It was because he underwent surgery for cochlear implants in order to try to restore some of his hearing, and the parents were told that if a ball ever hit him in the head, the surgery might have to be redone.

It had been seven years since Colin played ball in the WPRD league. I learned that in the intervening years, few youngsters with visible impairments of any kind had played in the sports leagues sponsored by the department. Many players were said to be taking Ritalin for their Deficit Hyperactivity Disorder (ADHD), and others had asthma. But as for youngsters with developmental, sensory, or more pronounced learning or behavioral disabilities, participation was rare.

Ray, a man who had coached for several years in the WPRD leagues, told me he had never encountered any other types of disabilities but had three boys who were taking Ritalin for their ADHD on the team he coached the year prior to the study. All the parents volunteered the information to him about their kids being on medication, but none of them offered any advice or guidance on how to deal with the boys' behavior. In his opinion, no one expected him to modify his program or offer them any special supports. Two of the boys did fine, but he found the behavior of the third boy intolerable. He missed a lot of practices, and when he did come to practices or games, he was very defiant and uncooperative. When he was playing centerfield on one occasion, he deliberately let a ball go by him (in Ray's opinion) without making a play for it. When Ray let the parents know he was feeling frustrated in dealing with the boy, the parents pulled him off the team, along with his brother (who had not presented any problems).

Mostly Asthma and Allergies

During the year of the study, 76 teams played in the WPRD summer baseball and softball leagues. I briefly examined approximately 600 enrollment cards for the girls and boys whose families registered them for these leagues. The cards did not ask about disabilities or special needs but did ask, "Does your child have any allergies or take any medication that his/her coach should be aware of?" Between 20 and 25 mentioned asthma; some added more specific comments such as, "carries her own inhaler." A few others identified allergies to specific drugs: penicillin, sulfa drugs, amoxicillin.

A small fraction of parents wrote in additional information or requests on the cards. Some were volunteering their help as coaches or assistant coaches. About 10 asked that the child not be assigned to the same coach as the previous summer. Drew explained that in most cases, this type of request stemmed from a personality conflict between the coach and the parent, not from any individual need of the child.

Only one parent identified the diagnosis of ADHD on the registration card (but didn't specify if the boy was on any medications); Drew assured me there were quite a few more who had ADHD, but whose parents didn't volunteer the information. One mother requested a coach who was "older and experienced" for her 12-year-old. The boy turned out to be Billy Walls, whom I met later; he was in special education and on Ritalin for ADHD. However, he never did show up for any of the baseball team practices or games, possibly because he knew his family was getting ready to move out of the area.

The mother of 16-year-old Sean provided the information that he was taking medications for seizures. Drew knew Sean and told me he was a very good athlete whose epilepsy had never interfered with his participation in sports. I arranged to meet him and his mom one day, just before his team took the field for a game. Youth who were still play-ing competitive baseball at age 16 were generally fit and better-than-average athletes, and by looks, Sean was no exception. He was solidly built and could have passed, based on physical size and bearing, for a college student. Only the braces on his front teeth betrayed his age.

After speaking with him, I watched him stroke a solid single through shortstop his first time up and then steal second base. He and his mom told me that he had his first seizure at age 12 and that he had only had three or four since. He didn't consider it in any way a drawback to his playing sports and certainly did not expect any modifications in rules or techniques for his benefit. However, he did always make sure his coaches knew about his condition.

The most important practical consequence of his seizure disorder that Sean could think of was that he would not be able to get a driver's license so long as he had to be on medication for the seizures. If he went without seizures and without medication for a certain period of time, then he would be able to drive.

Sean's case was thus the exception that proved the rule: Youth with any kinds of special needs that interfered in substantial ways with their athletic abilities were rarely joining WPRD sports teams. As a result, there was very little need for the coaches or those in charge of the leagues to consider any forms of modified participation in order to make the leagues more inclusive.

Joining a Team with Younger Peers

One approach the WPRD took to the inclusion of youth with dis-abilities on the infrequent occasions when their parents did register them for the baseball leagues was to have them play on teams with younger children. This concept had evolved over the years, originating in requests the department had received from parents whose children had no special needs. These families wanted their children to "play up" or "play down" (i.e., be assigned to a team with children one or more years older or younger than they were), either because they thought their children had sufficient athletic talent to compete with older chil-dren or insufficient talent to keep up with their peers. Such requests had been made frequently enough that a set of department guidelines had been developed.

Drew explained the guidelines as follows: If the parents wanted their youngster to play up one league, the request was automatically ap-proved. But if the parents wanted a child to play down, it was judged on a case-by-case basis. Department managers found that the former requests came in circumstances where children had already been playing ball with older siblings or more advanced youth and were simply ready for stiffer competition than they would find at their own age level. They saw no reason to second-guess the parents' preferences.

Parental requests to play down, on the other hand, were viewed with a more wary eye. The hesitation to accept all such requests at face value was captured by Drew's characterization of them as requests for "red-shirting." (Red-shirting refers to the practice of keeping athletes eligible for competition in high school or college for an extra season by holding them back before they begin their first year of eligibility.) As Drew explained, the WPRD did not want to allow parents to hold back a child to enhance his or her ability to dominate the opposition through greater strength, coordination, or maturity.

In order to prevent what they regarded as the misuse of the playing down option in baseball and softball, the managers had written into the official department rule book two conditions: (a) Children playing below their age level were not allowed to be pitchers; (b) These children also could not be selected for an all-star team. These conditions, Drew believed, operated as disincentives to any families who may have been tempted to use the playing down option as a form of red-shirting.

Assigning Children with Special Needs to Younger Teams

Drew added that in the cases where there was a special need or developmental issue that occasioned the preference for playing down, the parents didn't expect the child to be a pitcher or an all-star, so the two special conditions had never been viewed by parents as handicapping their children's participation. I also learned that in rare instances, a child (with or without special needs) was moved down one league not because of a parental request but at the initiative of a coach. I spoke with one coach who had a girl with learning disabilities on his team. After observing the child at the first two practices, he concluded she would do better in a league with younger girls. He spoke to the parents and, with their consent, arranged for her to be reassigned to a younger team.

I found this question of how to assign players who were not athletically on a par with their peers to be worthy of greater reflection than it appeared to have received within the department. A request for a child to play with younger participants (or with older ones) was a statement that individual differences in children's abilities had to be taken into account; that is, that one-size-fits-all policies that looked only at age as a factor were sometimes inadequate. A department that recognized this fact, it seemed, had grasped one of the values that underlay the principles of inclusion. Yet having grasped that value, was the only possible adjustment to leave the age-based leagues intact and reassign individual players who were viewed as developmentally (or at least, athletically) anomalous?

Was there a danger that it could be demeaning to a child with special needs to be put on a team with younger participants? In previous generations, children and adults with special needs were often put into groups without regard to their individual needs or interests. (Young children were placed with adolescents, for instance, or adolescents were grouped with middle-aged adults.) For this reason, advocates of inclusive opportunities have strongly encouraged that children with disabilities be kept with typically developing peers of the same age whenever possible.

Among a series of questions suggested in one book to determine if an agency is committed to inclusive practices is the following: "Are participants enrolled in programs that are chronologically age-appropriate, reflecting participation in the type of activities typical of the referent age group without disabilities?" (Weiss, Rynders, and Schleien 1995, 15).

If we asked this question about the participation of a child with special needs on a baseball team with younger players, we could answer with some confidence that the activity is indeed age-appropriate. (It is a long stretch from playing on a team with children two or three years younger than oneself to an example that Walker [1994] gives of an age-inappropriate activity: an adult with disabilities who plays with stuffed animals.) Furthermore, assignment to a different age group—at least as I observed it in the WPRD leagues—was based on a recognition of *differing abilities* but was not rooted in labels, assumptions, or preconceptions about *disabilities*. If the goal was to place the child in a league that would allow the closest match with the athletic prowess of his or her teammates, the solution adopted seemed to be reasonable. One question it overlooked, however, was whether in certain instances, children (or their families) might prefer for social reasons to have teammates of the exact same age, even if they performed at a conspicuously lower level of athletic ability.

From my limited view, the playing down option did seem largely beneficial. Lindy's parents had spoken with pride of her experience playing softball with girls younger then she. During my research, I learned about another 12-year-old girl with mild mental retardation who played down one league. I do not count her as one of the 19 children I studied in depth because I was never able to make contact with her father, a single parent. I watched her briefly in the field and at bat. She had less social interaction with her teammates—a very chatty bunch of 9- and 10-year-olds when they were on the bench—than most of them had with each other. However, her developmental differences were not very apparent in her on-field performance. I was told by an adult who knew her and her family that she was much happier this season (and getting on base a lot more often) compared with the previous summer when she had competed against girls her own age.

Selecting an Understanding Coach

One other tool available to Drew when a child with special needs registered to play on a team was to take a hand in the selection of the coach to which the boy or girl would be assigned. He was proud that his department did not allow coaches to select their own players, as was commonplace in many leagues. As he described the practice in other leagues, players were given an opportunity to display their talents at a mass tryout, and then coaches took turns choosing the ones they wanted on their teams. In Wabash, the WPRD staff made the assignments themselves for all the Wabash players. (Those from other towns were recruited and organized into their own teams through a separate process.) This gave Drew and his co-workers the ability to spread among different teams the youth they knew to be the most athletically talented and to make sure that players with poor attendance records in the previous season (as he explained) didn't all end up on the same team. In the case of a child who might need extra attention or instruction, this system allowed Drew to select a coach he thought would be sensitive to the child's individual needs.

The only time Drew told me that he might not want to be quoted (making a gesture toward the notepad on which I was scribbling as we sat in his office) was when he explained that he didn't assign children with special needs randomly. His understanding of his obligation under the law was that he should treat a child with a disability exactly the same as any other. But when he knew a child had special needs, he said, "I'm not going to just give him to any coach, and the coach I'm going to choose is not going to be one that I don't know. It's going to be one that I know." He asked the coach in such cases to keep him posted and let him know if there were any problems. "Maybe I shouldn't admit this. But that's what I do." He seemed to be fearful that this conscious effort to ensure the child's success could be viewed as a form of discrimination.

In actuality, the nondiscrimination provisions of both the ADA and its predecessor, Section 504 of the Rehabilitation Act of 1973, encouraged the kind of active solicitation of the well-being of the person with disabilities that Drew was practicing. Both laws required covered programs to make reasonable and readily achievable modifications in order to ensure access and participation to individuals with disabilities. The WPRD was subject to section 504 as a recipient of federal dollars and to the ADA as an agency of municipal government. Selecting an experienced coach who could be counted on to be fair and understanding of the individual with disabilities certainly would easily fall within the concept of a reasonable modification (if indeed it needed any legal justification at all), one that would not stigmatize the child and, moreover, one that could be critical to his or her successful participation.

TWO WHO DIDN'T PLAY BALL

The fear that their children might find themselves stigmatized or ostracized led two Wabash mothers I interviewed to steer sons who had mild physical disabilities away from organized team sports as a leisure-time option. Their names did not appear on the cards I searched through—but not because of any lack of interest in baseball.

Twelve-year-old Henry Watson's cerebral palsy had given rise to fine motor, gross motor, and language delays when he was younger, but thanks to early intervention, several years of therapy (through kindergarten) and the maturation process, his only remaining deficits were in gross motor development. It took him to age nine to learn to ride a bicycle; he had not yet managed to swim, according to his mother.

Finding an Alternative Sport

When I met Henry, he told me he liked to play basketball, but his mother told me that he had also had a very unhappy experience with the school basketball team. She and her husband had decided to let him try out, knowing it would be hard for him.

And he did not make the A team. There's also a B team; he was on that one, but he only played once or twice. By the end of the season, he came home really upset. We said, "that's OK," we gave him a hug, and tried to say, "OK, you didn't make a bucket, but I can't make a bucket either!" And, "if you want to try again next year . . ." And he says, raising his voice, "No, I'm not!" So, we said, "you may feel that way for now . . . let's see how you feel next year."

Meanwhile, they looked for an activity that would allow him to be part of a group and to compete but not to be in a situation where his motor problems could be viewed as detracting from the achievements of the other members of the team. They felt that they (and he) had found this in karate, which he took up with great enthusiasm. That experience is discussed in a later chapter.

Protecting a Son from Embarrassment

Tara—the mother of Brett, a third-grade boy with mild cerebral palsy, and married to Ray, the coach of three boys with ADHD mentioned earlier in this chapter—was even more leery than Henry's parents of the competitive sports arena. She admitted she was somewhat protective of her only child. When his cerebral palsy was diagnosed at the age of two, the internist who made the diagnosis told her (as mentioned in an earlier chapter) that he would use a wheelchair for the rest of his life. She felt fortunate that this prediction had turned out to be completely erroneous. (With physical therapy, he was walking six weeks later, without braces or any equipment.) But his gait had never been normal: His foot turned in, and he got pain in one hip when he walked any distance. He also had some visual problems.

Tara signed him up for Tiger Cubs and then Cub Scouts, in first and second grade—and was pleasantly surprised at how easily he was accepted by the other boys. But she feared the kinds of comments and reactions that might arise if he tried to join a baseball team.

Ray did not share her stance on this point. They were a blended family, and they both saw that Brett had benefited from being around Ray's son, Ray junior, who was three years older than Brett and spent a lot of time with him. "One of the best things," Ray said, "was getting around Ray junior, wrestling, bending his legs . . . he can run now, and he can fall down and brush it off. He used to scream for his mom if he fell down."

"I was overprotective," she acknowledged. They both felt that Brett's movements were much less stiff and more elastic now that he had engaged in rough-and-tumble play with his stepbrother. In addition to Cub Scouts, Brett had in the past two years tried and enjoyed water slides, roller-skating, and horseback riding.

They told me that, influenced by Ray junior's enthusiasm for baseball, Brett was watching more baseball and wanted to be on a team. Because of his interest, his parents were trying to figure out how to respond. "What I won't say to him," Tara said, "is what I think, which is that it will be really frustrating to him." She went on:

What I say instead is, it's a big commitment. You have to go to all the practices, and there's a certain number of games, and since you go to see your dad in the summer, it's not fair to the team to say you're only going to be on the team up to a certain point and then you're going to take off.

But really how I feel is, it will be a bad experience. And I guess I'm going to have to come up with a different response, because when he came back this last time from visiting with his dad, he said, "next summer I can go in August, I don't have to miss baseball."

While Tara was thinking about what kind of rationale to use to keep him from a potentially unsuccessful experience, Ray was advocating for a different approach. Having been a coach in the WPRD leagues himself, he knew that they could request for Brett to play down one league. "It will be a good learning experience," Ray said. "If he's playing against younger kids, he still might not excel, but it would keep him from appearing completely inadequate. Let him find out for himself if he can play well enough, and let him make up his own mind if he wants to continue."

Tara, who had heard this argument before but wasn't convinced, replied, "I guess I'm looking at it from a mother's point of view." One thing they both did agree on was that if they allowed Brett to join a team as he said he wanted, he would be required to stick it out for the whole season.

The discussions with the parents of Henry and Brett helped to illuminate the thinking of parents who must make decisions for (and together with) their children who had mild disabilities. Their perspectives helped to clarify why I found so few youth with special needs playing on WPRD teams.

ONE WHO PLAYED TEE-BALL

Carlton, a seven-year-old boy with developmental delays, played on a tee-ball team during the year of the case study. (Tee-ball is a version of baseball, in which batters do not attempt to hit a pitched ball but swing at a soft ball that sits on a metal tee that supports the ball at about the height of their waists.) With the permission of his foster family and the two women who coached the team, I took on the role of assistant coach, replete with baseball mitt and team T-shirt, in order to gain as thorough an understanding as possible of his experiences and the perceptions of those most closely involved with him.

Carlton was playing down one league: Tee-ball was advertised for five- and six-year-old boys and girls. Seven- and eight-year-old boys played in a league in which coaches pitched to their own players, and girls that age played in coach-pitched softball. (Carlton did not turn seven until nearly the end of the season but that still made him a seven-year-old in the eyes of the WPRD leagues, which used a player's age on August 1 as his age for the season.)

Tee-ball: Promoting Learning, Not Competition

The WPRD promoted the tee-ball league as a learning experience, avoiding the pressure of competition that tended to engulf the leagues to a greater degree as children aged and moved up through the different leagues. As they played it, runs scored were not recorded, meaning there were no winners and no losers. Each child played the field in every inning (adding extra infielders or outfielders if necessary), and each player batted once every inning, without respect to the number of players on the team. Moreover, each player trotted down to first base after hitting off the tee and stayed on as a base runner, even in the rare instances when the opponents caught the ball on the fly or threw successfully to make the out at first base. Each base runner advanced one base with each successive batter. When the coaches announced "last up!" every half-inning, that was the signal to let runners advance all the way across home plate. The lucky batter who occupied the last spot in the batting order had the thrill of hitting a home run in every inning of the entire game—or at least rounding all the bases as if he or she had done so.

All these measures were designed to lessen the importance of ability differences and reduce the performance pressure on these five-and six-year-olds, some of whom would not even attend kindergarten until after their first tee-ball season. The idea was that children could practice their skills and improve their knowledge of the rules and protocols of the game without the fear or frustration associated with winning and (especially) losing.

Thus, tee-ball (at least its Wabash version) seemed ready-made to ease the way for the participation of a child with special needs and remove the barriers that caused the parents of Henry, Brett, and possibly others to steer their youngsters away from team sports. A close examination of Carlton's tee-ball season not only illuminates how tee-ball in Wabash did, indeed, accommodate one child with developmental differences rather easily but can help probe the reasons why such differences may not be so readily accommodated among older age levels.

Carlton's History and Special Needs

Carlton and his biological sister, Darcy, who was one year older, were from Brewster and had been in foster care for a year and a half with a family in Wabash when I met them and their foster parents. Both children received special education services, and both were going to be in first grade in the year following the tee-ball season (she to repeat it, and he for the first time). As I was completing this writing, the two children were increasing their visitations with their biological mother in Brewster and preparing to go back with her full-time. Darcy attended a Brownie troop that I observed and that is discussed in a later chapter.

Steve and Sheila, the foster parents, also had two teenaged biological children plus an adopted nine-year-old and a baby boy whose adoption became final during the study. They explained that Carlton was labeled by the state agency responsible for his foster care placements as having cerebral palsy.[1] However, from studying the medical record themselves, the foster parents believed there were questions about this, because the diagnosis was made at age 20 months, after he had been abused in a previous foster placement. Whether his special needs originated from a congenital disorder or were attributable to brain injury inflicted on him during his younger years, the disabilities that he displayed included hemiplegia (spasticity on one side of the body), ADHD, and a seizure disorder. Carlton also had come to Steve and Sheila with speech and language delays and had speech therapy for the first year he was with them. But after making good progress in that area of development, speech therapy was discontinued. I found he used language competently, if less frequently and fluidly, than a typical child of his age.

Carlton wore a plastic brace on his right leg, from the knee to the ankle, and favored that side as he walked or ran. The brace was visible in the summertime, as he usually wore shorts, including during the tee-ball practices and games. He used his left arm as much as possible; for instance, wearing his baseball glove on the left hand, then taking it off after he caught or picked up a ball and throwing with the same arm. He batted off the tee from the right side, however, leaning with most of the weight on the left leg and using mostly his left arm as he stepped parallel to the tee and swung the bat. When one of the coaches reached out to give him a handshake at one point, reaching with her right toward his right hand, I saw him instantly retract that hand and substitute the left.

Parental Perspective on Recreational Activities

Sheila was a full-time homemaker, while Steve worked for the town of Wabash. She said the idea to sign Carlton up for a baseball team came naturally, when she saw how much he enjoyed playing ball in the yard with her older boys. From what she understood of his physical developmental needs, throwing, batting, and running bases would all be good for Carlton. She also said, "I wanted him in there for the social skills . . . and to help him fit in with other kids. He has problems not being like the other kids."

Even though she stated that she thought he would benefit from a recreational opportunity with typically developing peers, she did not sign him up for the WPRD league until she had first investigated the Special Olympics, which held its activities in Brewster. What she learned was that their softball teams were only for those aged 16 and up; they would let him come for practices in track and field events, if he wanted, but he couldn't actually be a competitor in that sport until he reached the age of eight. She thought going to practices and being excluded from competitions would "make him feel worse." That's when she turned to the WPRD.

Later in the summer, he attended an Easter Seal Society sleepover camp an hour away, a special camp that had different weeks for youth with various types of disabilities. (He attended the week for those with physical disabilities.) Sheila (like Lindy's mom) seemed interested in exposing him to a variety of recreational experiences and did not place greater value on either an inclusive or a "special recreation" model of services.

Assignment to League and Team

The decision for Carlton to play down, if he were going to join a league with typically developing peers, was one about which Sheila felt strongly. From the church she attended, she knew the woman who was Drew's assistant at the WPRD, the staff member who spoke with most parents when they stopped by the WPRD office to register their youngsters. She went in and spoke with her, telling her that Carlton was only "in the twentieth percentile for height, and emotionally young for his age." Could they have permission to put him in tee-ball instead of the coach-pitched league for seven- and eight-year-old boys? The assistant spoke with Drew and then told her Carlton would be permitted to play down.

Unsure of the nature of Carlton's disabilities, or whether they were of much consequence, Drew decided to assign him to a team on which his wife Tracy, was going to be the assistant coach (and on which their son would play). The lead coach, Rhonda, was a physical education teacher in the Wabash elementary schools. Rhonda told me she had been contacted by Drew before he finalized the assignment. This was consistent with the way Drew had described his handling of coaching assignments in cases where children were known to have special needs. He had given her the little information he had and asked her if she would be comfortable working with this boy (at this stage, the child's name was not used).

According to Rhonda, she had asked only one question. "I asked how tall he was. I was just thinking, if he was a head taller than everybody else, it would be hard for him to fit in and be accepted. But Drew surprised me by saying, 'Well, nobody is going to accuse you and Tracy of red-shirting!' Believe me, that wasn't even on my mind!"

When Rhonda saw an earlier draft of this book manuscript containing her quotation, she added this comment in writing: "I didn't want Carlton to feel out of place; I didn't worry about what the other children would think." (She was confident the other kids would accept him.)

Once she and Tracy agreed to have the boy on their team and were given his name, Rhonda then telephoned a physical education teacher she knew at the school that Carlton attended. "She said he tries anything. There was no problem with motivation; if you tell him to do something, he'll do it."

When Tracy telephoned to inform Carlton's family about the practice schedule (as she did with all the players' families), Sheila told her a little about his disabilities. It was the first time she or Rhonda learned that he had a diagnosis of cerebral palsy. Sheila told me that Tracy was very accepting, assured her that she and Rhonda were not worried about his participation at all, and did not press her for any details about his special needs, beyond what she volunteered.

Managing Carlton's Behavior and Supporting His Growth

Did Sheila and Steve want the coaches to cut Carlton some slack in light of his developmental delays? No. In fact, she told me during an in-

terview with the two of them together that "they should push him . . .
he needs to be pushed."

At the first practice I attended (it was the second one for Carlton), I
observed several instances in which his attention span seemed to be
much shorter—or his inclination to comply with instructions much
less—than any of the other players. Rhonda and Tracy divided the kids
into small groups to practice throwing and catching, fielding grounders, and hitting off the tee. Carlton was the only one who flitted away at
times from his assigned group—and without saying anything to the
coaches. He was also the only one who asked in the middle of practice
to go to the bathroom. On two different occasions, he abandoned the
practice routines to begin running the circuit of the bases, as if he had
just hit a home run. He seemed to be having fun; Tracy and Rhonda encouraged him to rejoin them but did not try hard to rein him in.

At the last practice before the opening game, Carlton sat down on
the field. Then he looked at me. (I was in my assistant coaching role,
wearing a glove and assisting in throwing and catching balls.) He asked
me for help in getting up. I asked him if he had pain, and he answered
yes. Tracy, who had overheard the interaction, then said something to
Steve who was watching from behind the backstop. Steve told her we
should ignore his complaints and tell him to get up and play. That's
what Tracy did.

After the first game, Sheila remarked on Carlton's tendency to move
in front of the protective backstop fencing while teammates were batting. She viewed this as a product of his ADHD, and the only real concern she ever expressed about his playing on the team was this one. She
wanted us to make sure he stayed behind the backstop and out of the
range of foul balls or thrown balls while other players were batting.
(Tee-ball is played with a rubberized ball, but a direct hit could still be
painful.)

At the end of a game or practice, Sheila or Steve often spoke casually
with Tracy, Rhonda, or me, updating us on aspects of Carlton's condition or disabilities. They told us about changes in his medications that
were made after he had a seizure at the beginning of the season. After
one of the first games, Sheila suggested to the coaches that Carlton
should be encouraged to bat left-handed rather than right-handed,
since that was his strong side and he may have to learn to bat from that
side as he gets older. "Last year," she explained, "one of the therapists
said it was important for him to work bilaterally." This year, she said she
was getting a different message: "He never will have much going in his
right arm, so just work with the left."

She referred to "constant disagreements" among the physical therapists (PTs) that worked with him over the past year. The one at the clinic they took him to in Brewster said one thing, she reported; the PT at school said another. (On top of that, there was a dispute over who was to pay for PT services. In accordance with the Individuals with Disabilities Education Act, school districts are responsible for therapies if and only if they deem them essential to the child's educational progress—and write them into the child's IEP.) "I've never had a doctor to go to who's known him since birth," she lamented, contrasting that to the situation with her biological children. She felt she was on her own, more so than with her other children, in trying to figure out what was best for him.

Focusing on the Game, Learning the Routines

Few of the other six boys and three girls had any head start on Carlton when it came to knowledge of the game. One of a series of general baseball knowledge questions Rhonda posed to the team as they sat on the ground, holding a brief team meeting after an early practice was, "Where's third base?" Only about half could point to it with great confidence.

In one game, in which our opponents were sponsored by (and were called) the Police, Ben, one of our most athletically inclined boys, stood at first base, rooting loudly for the other team. Apparently it was because he admired policemen.

Kimberly, while catching grounders at an early practice, removed her mitt, then asked, "Can I take this off? My hand is sweaty." "No," Rhonda answered, "you have to put it back on. Please—put it on." Later in the season, still suffering from the heat, Kimberly would tell me she wished our uniforms could be tank tops.

In my field notes after game one I wrote: "Although Carlton wandered more than anyone else, it was in ways that looked less divergent than in practice. He was the only child on either team who had to leave during the one-hour game to go to the bathroom, but he went with his mom to the park in the adjacent block while our team was on offense and without missing his turn in the batting order."

The following is taken from notes I wrote after game two: "Carlton is able to blend in pretty well, although he had to leave third base for a bathroom break when he was a base runner and sat down at his position in outfield around third inning."

In the games, in contrast to the early practices, Carlton stayed re-markably close to his assigned fielding positions (all players rotated through all positions over the course of the season, staying in a single position throughout any given game). He managed to avoid behaviors that would have made him look conspicuous to a casual observer. Throughout the season, he never ran off the field while we were on de-fense or tried to bat when it wasn't his turn or took off to run the base paths as he had in that early practice. When a hit ball landed near him, he was as good as any of the team at giving it a heave in the general di-rection of first base.

Proficiency with Glove and Bat

In game four, I noticed that Carlton stopped bringing his glove out to the field at all. This was sensible, in a way, given that he always re-moved it to throw and didn't really know how to catch with it (a skill that his teammates had not developed yet either). Then, in game eight (the last one he attended), he wore it for the first time on his right hand, as a left-hander should. It played a purely decorative purpose, as he picked up balls with his bare left hand. No one had instructed him to do this; evidently, he was beginning to assimilate knowledge through his own observations.

With or without his glove on either hand, Carlton paid reasonably good attention to the action throughout the season. By contrast, Kim-berly, while playing third base in game four, tried to sit down. Later, she covered her face (while still playing the field) with a rain slicker.

I tried to count the number of misses that Carlton made when bat-ting off the tee and compare them with Ben, our slugger, and with Kim-berly, one of our weaker hitters. It was difficult to keep the count precisely in my head while I was helping to keep the batting line-up in order, set the ball on the tee, and cheer on the squad. I noted the fol-lowing after game two: "Hard to tell who's weak, who's strong; for ex-ample, Ben actually missed more than Kimberly, although he hit farther—like Babe Ruth?" After game four I wrote: "I counted that Carlton missed three or four before making hit in first at bat; next at bat he had two misses, two that dribbled short of the chalk circle, and once hit the post before connecting. This is a little worse than other players but not so dramatic as to be noticeable. Even the sluggers like Ben do hit the post or miss the ball."

It seemed to me and the coaches that, with experience, his ability to focus was slowly improving. His parents, however, thought some of the improved focus that we observed was due to changes in the types and amounts of medication he was taking. These adjustments were made twice during the season, in the aftermath of a seizure he had just a few days prior to game one.

Social Interaction

The amount of peer interaction among all the players was minimal, all season, but I did observe Carlton interacting more with his teammates at the last game he attended than ever before. I also saw him speak with a child on the opposing team, something he had never done before. He told me that he knew the boy from Bible camp.

One observation was consistent from his first game to his last: He loved it when his teammates, standing behind the backstop, chanted his name when he came up to bat. This chanting for the batter was an activity I had initiated, and it was born of necessity on the spur of a moment. The tee-ball diamonds were very spare; there were no benches for players or bleachers for family members. Spectators arrived—and there was a good turnout—with blankets and lawn chairs. When the team came in from the field, each player knew he or she would have a turn to bat, so they had nowhere to go except to crowd around the backstop, anxiously awaiting their turns. Rhonda had given me the job early on of keeping the players lined up in the proper order. To keep them focused on the game, I encouraged them to chant for the batter, and many of them did it with enthusiasm. My field notes after game one stated: "When they [chanted his name], he beamed a bigger smile than I'd seen on any kid all evening. They had put the accent on the second syllable: 'Carl-tin! Carl-tin! Carl-tin!' Maybe that support was what helped him to belt one so hard! He always needs a reminder to start running, though."

In his last game, I again observed that he beamed when he heard his own name chanted. But I also noted for the first time that he took part in the chanting of other teammates' names and seemed to enjoy it.

I never saw any evidence that Carlton's peers considered his behavior to be different, his skills to be deficient, or thought his leg brace was noteworthy. Rhonda had twin girls who played on the team. She asked them after the season was over whether they had noticed anything different about any of the players, that would mean that someone "had a handicap or special needs" of some kind. They had not.

Inconsistent Attendance

Carlton missed five games in a 10-game season. He missed the final two games and the team cookout while attending an Easter Seal Society special camp for kids with physical disabilities. He was absent for one practice and the taking of the team photograph a few days before the first game because he had a seizure one afternoon at school and had to be rushed to a hospital in Brewster. (He was hospitalized overnight and his seizure medication was changed.)

He missed three other games in a row, in midseason. According to his mom, she and Steve lost track of the schedule for two of the three games that he missed. They missed the other one because of preparations for the final steps toward adoption of another foster child—an adoption that was considered newsworthy due to their association with an innovative foster care agency. Journalists and photographers demanded their time in connection with this.) She was an enormously busy parent with her six children. Steve's job working for the municipality of Wabash often kept him busy into the evening hours (tee-ball was held on week nights from 6:00 to 7:00 P.M.). In sum, I interpreted their losing track of the tee-ball schedule neither as a product of disinterest nor of a disorganized household but as a by-product of their multifaceted commitments. Some of these commitments were those that any parent in a large family faced, others were those of a parent whose child had special needs (subject to such unpredictable events as a seizure), and still others distinctively those of a family with a conscious commitment (through foster care and adoption) to care for more than one child with special needs.

Although his absences require no justification, Carlton's attendance record is worth pondering as we consider the challenge facing coaches and leagues such as those of the WPRD that are trying to promote inclusion of youth with disabilities. The majority of the 10 players on the team missed at least one game (because of chicken pox and family vacations, for instance) but only one other missed as many as three. No one else missed the final game and the cookout. I made this note after the final game:

The kids developed a lot more peer interaction by the end of the season. While in line to bat, they actually had dialogue on such things as whether this was the last game, would there be a snack in addition to the cookout, where to leave your mitt between innings.

Also, more of them were making better contact with the ball in hitting. And the throwing was improved, but little evidence for being able to catch a ball, thrown or hit.

Carlton is in Easter Seal camp this week, but it looks like by missing games, he missed the skill development and social development.

To compensate for his physical and social deficits, it would have been beneficial for Carlton to be present at least as consistently as his teammates. Yet, for perfectly legitimate reasons, he attended fewer practices and games than anyone else.

In a joint interview with Rhonda and Tracy after the season ended, Rhonda commented on the absences:

Carlton was coming late. Like the day it was his turn to play first base, he didn't get there on time. And then he was missing games. I think if you have special needs, it's even more important to be on time, to make sure they hear what goes on at the beginning. If you miss the beginning, you can be lost. And you also miss out on some of the camaraderie. Pitching the ball back and forth with someone before the game starts, going for a little jog. I would say this is something for parents to really think about.

It seemed to me that from the viewpoint of a volunteer coach (or a staff member like Drew), erratic attendance also complicated the process of determining the source of problems—if there were any. Did they stem from the child's disabilities? Or could they be attributed to the inconsistent attendance? I was reminded of Ray's comments about having three boys with ADHD on his team the previous season, two of whom blended in just fine with the team and one who did not. He had noted that the difficult boy was also the one who missed practices and arrived late for games. Perhaps the erratic attendance was as important as the ADHD in undermining the boy's ability to be successful.

MODIFICATIONS OF RULES OR PROCEDURES IN WPRD SPORTS LEAGUES

When Cliff, the boy who was hired to help with the tee-ball equipment, used to be on a baseball team, Drew told me he gave Cliff's parents a batting helmet to take home and customize. Ordinarily, a batter picked up any helmet as she or he headed for the on-deck circle; no advance planning was required. But because the helmets caused Cliff's hearing aids to whistle, Drew told his family they could take one home and "do whatever they needed to it" to outfit it properly for the boy's head.

This small illustration indicates that adaptations were not a completely novel concept in the WPRD sports leagues. It also illustrates that adaptations for youth with disabilities need not always be elaborate, expensive, or contingent on specialized training.

I did not come across any other examples of adaptations for children with disabilities in the WPRD baseball and softball leagues. I did, however, attend an interesting discussion about rule making and rule modifying during the orientation meetings for coaches. I learned that there was nothing sacrosanct about the WPRD league rules and that WPRD staff, in consultation with coaches, had revised them over the years. (The boys' leagues for players aged 13 and up were affiliated with national associations that had their own rule-making bodies. All other rules were under the jurisdiction of the WPRD.)

A portion of each orientation was devoted to making sure that all the coaches clearly understood the rules and an explanation for any rule that had been changed or modified. An example of a rule that had been changed was the one that determined when a 9- and 10-year-olds' team on offense had to stop batting, in the event the opposition was unable to get three outs. The general rule was that a team was limited to a maximum of 10 batters per inning, even if there were fewer than three outs. However, they had revised the rule in the last inning—only for the team that was trailing. In the event they were so far behind that application of the rule would make their winning a mathematical impossibility (i.e., if they were behind by more than nine), they could continue to bat until the other team got all three outs.

In the discussion, no one made reference to how rule changes might inhibit or promote the development of more inclusive leagues that would benefit those with disabilities. But it struck me that the rationale that Drew had presented—that the rules were not immutable, that league officials could change them to meet the needs of the players—was one that developers of inclusive recreation could also use to justify accommodations in rules or procedures for participants with disabilities.

INCLUSION IN MORE ADVANCED BASEBALL OR SOFTBALL LEAGUES

Neither of Carlton's tee-ball coaches saw much difficulty in Carlton, or a child with a similar level of special needs, playing in the coach-pitched league the next year or two. But neither saw (barring significant developmental advances) how Carlton would be able to compete in the player-pitched leagues that began when children turned nine. If he chose to play at all, they envisioned him relegated to the status of bench warmer.

"As soon as you keep score and have won and lost records," Rhonda said, "the learning goes out the door." Tracy agreed, adding that "the coaches don't bother trying to teach anything to the ones they look on as less developed."

Tracy talked about her own nephew, who had no special needs and this year became eligible for the 9- and 10-year-old league. She was surprised and dismayed at how few innings he was put into the games by his coach. Moreover, he was "always stuck in right field." Meanwhile, the better athletes "were never put in the outfield and never taken out of the game. . . . you'd think at least if the team is way ahead or way behind that's when they'd give a kid . . . a chance to try a different position."

Both of these women were strongly rooted in the local community. Tracy came from a farming family and had lived in Wabash her entire life. Rhonda had lived all but one year in Wabash. But they both seemed estranged from what they regarded as the predominant attitude toward competitive sports that prevailed in the town. Tracy, being married to Drew, was aware of the pressures that some parents tried to put on him; for instance, to make sure their boy or girl could be a pitcher. Both women viewed the whole climate toward competitive sports as unfortunate, not only for youth with special needs, but for the majority of youth who were not athletically gifted. For many of the same reasons, Rhonda preferred, in her professional life, to stick with elementary-aged, rather than high school-aged, physical education classes.

The competitive environment that they described was in contrast to the goals of the leagues as presented in two coaches' orientation meetings I attended before the season began. At these meetings, Drew distributed copies of three articles from *USA Today* and the Editorial Projects Department of *Sports Illustrated*, all of which made one central point in different ways: that the underlying purpose of the league was to help children have fun. Number 2 on a list of 10 quiz statements was this one: "It is important for children to learn how to compete at an early age." The correct response (out of three offered) was: "No. The earlier young children learn to be competitive, the less enjoyment they might have in playing."

In Palo Alto, California, a new baseball league, the Youth Baseball Athletic League (YBAL), was initiated in the 1990s, beginning from the premise that a huge number of youth drop out of organized sports between ages 12 and 14 because "they're not having fun, and they're turned off by abusive coaches.[2] In YBAL, every child played every inning, as in tee-ball, and there were no league standings.

Rhonda said she had heard of other leagues in other parts of the country at the local level that operated on those same principles. She told me that where her sister lived, in another midwestern state, there were noncompetitive recreational leagues that were available in some communities alongside the more traditional competitive leagues. She said she could not at present envision how the WPRD could change. "But I can see how some parents might step out of it and enroll their kids in a more recreational type program." She paused and added, "and I might be one of those that would do that."

5

The Youth Recreation Center: Many Drop In, One Family Opts Out

It was possible to imagine all the adults disappearing from the Youth Recreation Center (YRC) and activities still going on more or less as they normally did. The fact that you could shoot baskets, play Ping-Pong, eat a bag of potato chips, draw pictures, or listen to music at your own pace, and without staff members hovering over you, explained a large part of its appeal to many youth—especially boys—who fell within the social and developmental mainstream. At the same time, this free-flowing, unstructured ambiance accounted in some measure for the infrequent participation of children with disabilities or special needs. It also seemed to contribute to the underrepresentation of girls among the more active members.

The YRC operated seven days a week as a coeducational, facility-based, drop-in club-style program. (There were also sports camps, day camps, school parties, weekly junior and senior high nights, and classes such as ballet, tap dance, and martial arts scheduled at specific times.) The center was under the administration of the Wabash Parks and Recreation Department (WPRD), with some of its financial support provided by the local park district, a taxing body separate from the town. It was not affiliated with any national organization. Membership was available to all local youth, ages 7 through 15. The most active members were in the 9 through 12 age group.

LAYOUT AND FEATURES OF THE CENTER

The facility, acquired by the town of Wabash just three years prior to the study, was a solid, modern, single-story brick structure that appeared to be in a good state of repair and was unmarred by graffiti or any other obvious problems. The east side of the building consisted of a huge, undeveloped grassy area, where center members frequently played kickball or just hung around, gravitating in warm weather toward the one large shade tree that stood about 100 feet from the building. Beyond the grassy area was a modest set of bleachers overlooking a field that was used for soccer. Behind the center were basketball courts, and beyond that, an 18–hole public golf course, which was under the jurisdiction of the park district.

The center's staff office was situated at the strategic nerve center of the operation. A staff member working inside the office could watch children arriving through the double set of front doors or could turn around the opposite way to look through picture windows onto the gym, which took up the largest share of the building.

The gym, with its full-length basketball court, six basketball goals, and high, cavernous, acoustically challenging ceilings, was the area that drew the largest number of members for the longest periods of time. I watched junior high–aged boys enter the gym and never leave it (except for a snack or a bathroom break) until it was time to go home, and boys as young as seven stick with their basketball shooting for more than an hour. A few girls were usually sprinkled among the basketball players if they were shooting around, or playing a competitive game, such as one called Knock-Out. Actual pick-up games were an exclusively male activity. Girls (and sometimes the youngest boys) improvised activities along the folded-in bleachers that ran the length of the back of the gym; for instance, rolling a volleyball or basketball back and forth, or practicing dance or cheerleading steps.

The entry area between the office and the front door was carpeted and had two round tables set aside for quiet activities, such as coloring, playing with board games or action figures, or constructing with Legos. (You requested games and materials from the staff; they kept everything in a walk-in closet along with the athletic equipment.) Here, one was more likely to encounter girls than boys. In the same area with the tables were several comfortable, wooden-framed, cushioned armchairs, which children seldom chose to sit in, but which were used by staff as seating for misbehaving children when they were given a "time-out." (On more than half of my visits to the center, I observed staff members giving time-outs to one, two, or three youth. Members accepted and discharged these sanctions with only mild grumbling; I saw none of these situations escalate into confrontations. I saw one boy fall asleep after 10 minutes of a time-out and remain asleep, sitting in his chair, for at least 90 minutes.)[1]

There was a TV near the office, which I saw turned on only once. (Children had to ask permission to watch it.) During the time I was conducting the case study, a 125-gallon salt-water aquarium was installed a few feet from the staff office. Rowdy or careless behavior in its immediate vicinity was forestalled by a chain-link barrier, the kind you would find around a sculpture that was not to be touched in a museum.

In the very front of the building were two office-type rooms. One was the director's office; I never once saw him sitting at his desk, but the door was always wide open. "I leave it that way on purpose," he told me. "I want children to understand that you don't go in somewhere that doesn't belong to you. It doesn't matter if it's locked up or not. You respect other people's space and their things."

The second door led to the music room. It housed a small library (made up of books discarded by the local schools) and a piano, and was furnished with one table, chairs, and a good-sized portable stereo (boom box). This room, in theory, was available for youth who wanted to sit and read or do their homework. In practice, it was a hangout where as many as seven or eight girls listened to music, played cards or other games, and sometimes practiced their dancing. Children who wanted to enter this room had to ask for staff permission; once they entered, they could close the door and enjoy their private space. One female staff member told me approvingly, "They just want a place where they can get away from the boys."

Turning left after entering the front door led to a multipurpose room with a linoleum floor, large enough to run activities for 40 children. It could be closed off through the use of a built-in, portable partition. This room was not used much during the regular drop-in activities but was where specially scheduled classes and day camp activities were held. Admission to these activities (and payment, if there was any) was handled separately from membership in the YRC.

Through the carpeted area, opposite the multipurpose room, was a game area, featuring pinball, video games, pool and Ping-Pong tables, and foosball. For the Ping-Pong paddles and pool cues, the center charged children $1 per hour, except during special times when they were made available for free. The games that were coin-operated took quarters, and children could request change at the office. These machines were modestly popular among the boys: It was not unusual to see a group of four or five gathered around the pinball or video game as a peer tested his luck (or skill). But these gatherings never seemed to last more than 15 or 20 minutes; unless someone had a hot streak and won some free games, the supply of quarters was soon exhausted and the children headed off to find something else to do. Pool or Ping-Pong occupied small numbers of boys (almost never girls) for longer periods of time.

A snack bar was the remaining feature of the front of the building, with compact but comfortable seating in seven booths that seated four apiece. There was a small but full-service kitchen (where the summer lunch program was based) with a counter and wide window that opened onto the snack bar, and another counter and window that opened from the kitchen onto the gym. These windows were left open, but during the daily and summer drop-in program, food was not allowed anywhere besides the snack bar. Children could sit in the snack bar to eat snacks brought from home or could purchase snack and beverage items from the YRC. Frequently (at the center director's discretion), the center staff served free food, such as peanut butter and jelly sandwiches or even hot dogs or pizza. The director accumulated a budget for these items by recycling the cans that members purchased from the soft-drink machine. (He showed me a check for $85 from a recent recycling expedition and pointed out that if he waited until hot dogs were on sale for 49¢ a package, he could feed a child a hot dog on a bun for 10¢ to 15¢ each.) When food was made available for free, word spread rapidly, and even youth who were actively engaged in outdoor activities (especially those age 12 or under) found their way promptly to the snack bar. Only the adolescent boys heavily into basketball were imperturbable and immune to the scent of the free food.

As indicated in the above description, one saw mostly boys in the gym and the games area, mostly girls at the quiet-table activities and in the music room. Overall, staff agreed with my observation that there were about twice as many boys as girls in attendance at most times.

SOCIAL COMPOSITION OF MEMBERSHIP

As with other club-style programs, you had to be a member to enter, but the annual fee was set low enough to be affordable even by families with limited resources. In 1996, the fee was $20 per year for the first child in the family and $10 each for siblings. On weekdays during the summer, members (and anyone else who wanted to take advantage of it) got a free hot lunch, courtesy of the town's designation of the center as a site for the federally funded Child Care Food Program.

Few who wanted to patronize the facility were left out, because a local foundation funded by area businesses was established in 1992 for the specific purpose of making the programs of the local park district and WPRD available to economically disadvantaged youth. (More recently, the United Way also came on board as a funder.) The foundation paid for passes to the YRC for approximately 30 percent of its members.[2] Parents who wished to receive this benefit for their children visited the office of a social service agency situated in the town's only shopping plaza.

Total membership in YRC in 1996 was a little above 700, including a core of 50 to 75 who attended frequently. Daily attendance figures in the spring and fall, when the center was open from 3:00 P.M. to 7:00 P.M., ranged from about 25 to 65, usually somewhere near the middle of that range. During the summer, with children out of school and the center open all day, the daily numbers were usually from 80 to 100. Weekend attendance (all day on Saturdays and after 1:00 P.M. on Sundays) was typically in the range of 40 to 60, both during the summer and the school year. The building was large enough that it did not begin to feel crowded until there were at least 50 to 60 children present—provided they were spread out among the different areas.

The availability of free memberships for low-income youth definitely influenced the composition of the population at the YRC and brought its racial and socioeconomic mix more in line than other youth activities with the actual population of the town. As indicated in chapter 3, 24 percent of the students, grades kindergarten through eight, were African American (and another 3 percent, Hispanic), and 48 percent of the children were classified as living in low-income households. Roughly one-quarter to one-third of members attending the drop-in program at any given time appeared to be African American. Among the first 121 memberships acquired with foundation support in 1996, 41 percent went to Caucasian youth, 32 percent to African American, 2.5 percent to Hispanic, and another 24 percent to youth who were of racially mixed background or whose ethnicity was unknown to the person reporting this information to me. In all the other activities I observed, participation of African American youth was anywhere from 0 to approximately 15 percent, with the exception of the Brownie troop that is the main focus of a later chapter (where 3 of 10 girls were African American).

Although there was no monitoring or reporting of attendance at the drop-in program by type of membership (i.e., those paid by families vs. those paid by the foundation), it was clear that the more active participants at the YRC were drawn disproportionately from the less affluent families of the community and that the foundation support was a major factor in achieving this outcome. Lower income youth were only slightly more likely than more affluent peers to join the YRC. But once they joined, those from less affluent homes had fewer options for out-of-school activities and therefore were more likely to become frequent users of the center. Also, some parents viewed the drop-in program as an extremely inexpensive alternative to paying for child care for school-age youngsters.

MANAGEMENT, STAFFING, AND SUPERVISION OF THE FACILITY

The director of the YRC, whom I'll call Greg, was a balding, energetic man in his fifties. Greg, who had previously been park and recreation director in a community of about the same size in the next county, appeared to live his job as YRC director rather than to just work there. He usually was present seven days a week, keeping tabs on the operation. Moreover, he sought ways to immerse himself ever more in the lives of the youth of Wabash and to make his facility relevant to other stakeholders in the community, regardless of the increase it caused in his own workload.

He personally initiated and usually worked at junior high nights (Fridays during the school year) and high school nights (Saturdays). He handled many of the instructional and leadership duties involved in special sports camps and sports leagues, such as Tee-ball camp in the spring and soccer in the fall, both of which took place on Saturdays. He did all the purchasing and some of the food preparation and cooking for the summertime hot lunch program. He initiated a father-son foul-shooting contest the weekend before Thanksgiving, with turkeys awarded to the winners. During weekdays, when the center didn't open until 3:00 in the afternoon, he was often in and out of the local schools. Sometimes he was making arrangements for collaborative activities, such as the popcorn and roller-skating parties for honor roll students that he began hosting for each of the four elementary schools once each quarter. He supervised those parties himself, together with the teachers that arrived with 60 or so children. Other times he was huddling with a principal to get the facts behind a rumor of an altercation, news of which had come to him through the YRC members. Or he might be seeking resources. (The funds for the aquarium came mostly from funds donated by high school seniors.)

His efforts at good public relations (and good service to children) had definitely made an impression on the elementary school principal I interviewed. I had not even brought up the subject of the YRC, but was asking her for some general comments on the availability of recreational options for young people after they went home from school or during weekends and vacations. "I think if people knew what was going on at the Youth Recreation Center, they'd move here [to Wabash] just for that!" She went on to describe a roller-skating party the parent-teacher organization of her school had recently held there, a very successful multigenerational family event.

"Greg! He is just somebody special! He has this wonderful balance," she said, going on to say that "he wants everybody to have fun, but at the same time, someone who lets you know there are rules and you have to respect them." As an example of this blend of goodwill and discipline, she laughed about a sign posted by the coatrack of the YRC: words to the effect that if you failed to hang up your coat properly and it landed on the floor, you would owe Greg 25 push-ups before you got it back.

She described another gesture of Greg's that conveyed a mixture of warmth, respect, and sarcasm: On the day teachers returned from winter holidays, he sent flowers to every school, honoring the public school staff and welcoming them back (and implicitly acknowledging his gratitude to them for ending his obligation to provide extended hours of operation at the YRC).

Greg usually scheduled three staff members (including himself if he anticipated being there) to handle the supervision of the drop-in program; there were times when it was only two, and times when it was more than three. Thus the ratio of staff to members at most times was about 1:20 or 1:25. The other paid staff were mostly young men and women in their late teens and early twenties, with a strong affinity for (but not professional training in) sports and recreation. The exceptions to this were a couple of more mature women who had experience as cooks in public schools and who therefore could be counted on to help take charge of the summer hot lunch program. One of these also had experience as a Boy Scout leader. All the staff, like Greg himself, had strong ties within the local community. Two young men on the staff were brothers, part of a large African American family he greatly admired. One of the young men on staff was the son of one of the women on staff.

Greg strengthened the level of staffing and supervision by recruiting some youth who had recently aged out of the drop-in program as volunteers. He pointed out a 15-year-old who had been coming seven days a week and would soon be too old to attend. "I spoke to him about volunteering next year," he said. "Not every day, but maybe a couple days a week." The young man sounded interested. "And then, I may be able to pay him at times. And if he wants to join the adult fitness center [operated by the town], I can also get him a discounted membership." The young people he hired for a few hours a week were made welcome to come at any time, and, as Greg viewed it, whenever they were playing basketball with the members, they were helping to enforce proper conduct, acting as volunteer staff, whether or not they were formally designated as such.

Greg's management style was personal and informal. There were no staff manuals, formal orientations, or staff development activities to clarify expectations for how staff should carry out their responsibilities. He did not appear to provide much specific guidance as to how and where individuals were to deploy themselves in order to provide supervision during their assigned shifts. At least one person stayed in the staff office to monitor children arriving and signing in, and to answer the telephone. Members could go outside to play without staff accompaniment during nice weather, after signing in. However, if Greg noticed that more than a dozen to 15 children were playing outside, he might ask a staff member to station herself out there for a while. When there were large numbers of youth in the gym, there was usually—but not always—a staff member stationed there. Supervision of the front areas (game room, music room, tables) was generally handled by someone walking through from time to time, not by having anyone stationed there to keep watch.

Rules for children's conduct were posted: "Profane or abusive language will not be tolerated"; "No caps or gum allowed"; "Phones may be used to call parents only (3 minutes)." There was also a posted set of consequences for breaking a rule: For the first offense, you got a warning; second offense, you got a warning and a phone call to a parent; third offense, a phone call home, plus a letter that may stipulate a suspension for any of several periods of time. But as to any overall disciplinary philosophy or any nonpunitive responses to the misbehavior of members (such as redirecting a child, helping him or her to find a way of resolving conflicts in the future and so forth), there was nothing in print.

Greg described himself as "a roamer," always moving around while he was on duty: speaking with children, planning upcoming events and schedules with staff, doing maintenance tasks, responding to a question from a parent. There were no staff meetings. It seemed that Greg offered his own style of supervision and interaction as an example to other staff, perhaps believing that was more meaningful than sitting people down at a meeting or giving them a staff handbook. If plans and programs were discussed, it was on the fly, with Greg talking one-on-one with various staff members as he did his roaming.

A CHILD'S EXPERIENCE IN THE DROP-IN PROGRAM

On entry, a child headed straight to the office window for the required sign-in, including name, membership ID number, age, and time. (A step stool was always at the ready, as the majority of members could not reach the counter to sign in without the extra step up it gave them.) As they signed in, a staff member exchanged greetings from inside the office and in some cases passed on messages from parents that had come by telephone or requests that were left over from previous days. ("This text book was left here on Tuesday; somebody said it was yours.")

When children signed in, nothing was said to them about the activity choices. The available equipment or materials did not vary from one day to the next. Members knew—or learned, soon enough, by watching their more experienced peers—that they had the run of the place, and it was up to them to find or create an activity they enjoyed. Whatever they chose, there was no obligation to stick with it or to stay in an area; they could always drop it and move along to something else—provided they weren't being disruptive or creating some kind of scene that drew the attention of staff.

About half of the youth on any given day at the center arrived with at least one sibling. If the siblings were the same gender, they were likely to head to an activity area together. If they were brother and sister, they usually split up after signing in. The gym seemed to be the place where a child could most comfortably go, lacking a sibling or friend to play with, and fit in relatively easily. The other areas—games, music room, table activities—pretty much required having a friend to start playing.

Of course, a child could ask for a puzzle and work on it alone, but that rarely happened.

From my observations at the center, the vast majority of members did find something to do within a few minutes, either with a same-sex sibling they arrived with, a friend they'd been dropped off with, or another friend they'd encountered right away. Most stayed with the initial activity for at least a little while. Moreover, most members, throughout their time in the drop-in program, looked like they were socially connected with someone else that was involved in the same activity—although on the basketball court, specific one-to-one relationships were harder to perceive. The instances I saw in which children appeared isolated, disengaged, or disenchanted were few and did not last long.

YOUTH WITH SPECIAL NEEDS

Among the active users of the YRC during the period of the case study, there were no youth with obvious disabilities. However, as noted in an earlier chapter, of the roughly 270 children from kindergarten through grade eight who received special education services in the Wabash public schools, about two-thirds of them were classified as having learning disabilities, and another 10 percent or so, behavior disorders. These were disabilities that in many cases would not be readily apparent in a physically active, recreational setting. The staff at the YRC were quick to acknowledge their belief that many of the children they served had these kinds of special needs. They assumed that a substantial number were receiving some kind of special help or were attending special classes. But unless the child or parent volunteered the information, staff (including Greg) had no awareness of which children were special education students, nor, when they did learn of it, was it particularly important to them: There was no conscious attempt to customize the program or plan activities with this understanding in mind.

In the office during my first visit, Greg showed me a list with three names on it. These boys were only allowed to be in attendance when Greg was present, because other staff members had been "going nuts" trying to figure out how to deal with their aggressive behavior. (Each case, he said, was completely separate from the other two.) This was a new strategy they were trying for the first time. He had come to know through his informal contacts with public school staff that at least one of the three attended a "special class." He thought the class was for students with behavior problems, but it could have been for children with learning disabilities. He wasn't sure, and it wouldn't have made any difference in the approach that he and his staff used in coping with the boy's behavior.

Through my contacts with family members in Wabash, I learned of the special educational backgrounds of a few of the youth who regularly attended the YRC. Lucas, one of a family of four boys who regularly attended the drop-in program, was a 13-year-old who was in fifth grade and barely reading and writing. His mother was growing increasingly distressed that the schools had not been able to successfully diagnose and respond to his learning disabilities (although they agreed he had them). She had pulled him out of public school one year and tried him in parochial school in Wabash, but that had been an even worse experience for him, with a larger number of students in his classroom and fewer opportunities for special help. She felt that his participation at the YRC was one of the best things going for him, because he was able to compete successfully with peers on the basketball court, something he could not do in an academic arena. When I spoke to Greg and another staff member at the YRC who knew Lucas, they acknowledged they would not have known of his significant special education needs. They would not have known that his brother, who was one year younger, was surpassing him academically.

Ginny and Barry Riley were sister and brother, ages nine and six respectively, who came frequently to the center; they also had an older sister, Lucy, age 11, who was living in another state when I first met the family. Greg put me in touch with their mother because there had been a serious altercation involving Ginny. He stated that he had no knowledge of whether she was a special education student, he just knew that she could be a real handful and said that her mom was concerned about her. Greg and Ginny's mom agreed in separate interviews that she had "gone off," wild with fury, on at least two occasions.

When I met with Ginny's mom, she confirmed Greg's impression that she was indeed very concerned about her daughter's occasional outbursts. She informed me that Ginny was not in special education but had repeated second grade, in part because of her erratic behavior. One point that emerged strongly from the interview was that the mom was extremely impressed with Greg's style of discipline with her daughter. "He can get Ginny to look him straight in the eye, to listen. I don't get that. I get the rolling of the eyes, the sighing . . . And that's what every teacher that's ever tried to discipline her has gotten." It wasn't because Greg was a softy, she said, who would let her get away with things. "He tells her what the consequences will be, tells her if she gets herself to be unwelcome there, that will apply to the [town] swimming pool as well." She said maybe it was because Ginny didn't view Greg as an authority figure. When I repeated this back to Greg, he commented, "Good. I'm glad she feels that way."

I learned in my interview that Lucy, the older sister, was in special education and was moving to rejoin them in Wabash soon. The YRC staff later met Lucy, and so did I. Lucy was a friendly girl whose interactive style and demeanor were unremarkable. She did not present any behavioral challenges to them. She would never have been identified to me by the YRC staff as a child who they thought had special needs. Playing blackjack with her and some other girls in the music room one afternoon—the kind of one-to-one involvement that the center staff, given their ratio and supervision style, very seldom experienced—I observed that she could not add one-digit numbers, such as 8 + 4, in her head. She had to count them on her fingers.

A WABASH FAMILY THAT SOUGHT AN ALTERNATIVE

I met one Wabash family who had custody each summer of the husband's adolescent son, Artie, with Down Syndrome and two younger siblings. (During the rest of the year, they lived with their mother in another state.) I would eventually meet Artie and see that he was a boy of normal build, friendly disposition, and good physical coordination. As they told me, he had a sizable vocabulary (if limited for his age), but you had to get used to the way he pronounced his words; you might not understand much at first.

Artie had not had a good experience in his few visits to the YRC when he went there with his 15-year-old stepsister during the summer of 1995. (He was 14 at the time.) According to his stepmother, whom I'll call Charlotte, some of the youth there had teased him. The story Charlotte got from her daughter was that none of the adults had done anything about it, so on at least one occasion she (the daughter) had to "start screaming at the kids." When Charlotte spoke with a staff member who had been there, she claimed that they had stepped in and gotten the members to stop teasing. But in either case, Charlotte told her, "it doesn't help to simply make them stop without educating them. You have to be a role model, and you have to use it as a learning situation."

One staff member at the YRC—no older than 19 or 20 years of age—confirmed some of the details of this story, although I had not even asked about it. We were making conversation as he supervised the basketball playing in the gym. I told him of the general focus of my research, and he responded with his recollection of the same incident that Charlotte had previously described.

He didn't recall Artie's name, but the timetable, the description of the boy, and the fact that he was there with a teenaged sister (he didn't realize the girl was really a stepsister) were consistent. He remembered that other members had teased Artie. He also remembered that Artie was good at video games and enjoyed both pool and Ping-Pong. (I would soon have my own opportunity to confirm his observations of Artie's experience with the pool cue.) When no youngsters had stepped forward to play with Artie, he recalled that he had played these games with him. He also recalled that Artie had a strong personality ("a temper," he said).

Charlotte's conclusion regarding the YRC was that "they have some nice people who work there, but they are not trained as youth workers." In the summer of 1996, both parents were working full-time, and they needed a place to take Artie every day where he would be adequately supported and offered appropriate activities. Because of that single unpleasant experience the previous summer at the YRC, Charlotte and her husband did not consider the YRC a viable option, although it was open full-time and would have been very convenient. Instead, they ended up driving him, as well as his 13-year-old brother Curt and 9-year-old sister Karen, to the Boys and Girls Club, 15 miles away in Brewster.

What advantages did the Boys and Girls Club offer over the Youth Recreation Center in their eyes? Charlotte and her husband cited three major considerations: (1) its affiliation with a national organization; (2) the way the social groupings were structured; (3) what they perceived as a closer, more intensive style of supervision.

I observed Artie at the Boys and Girls Club in Brewster and at a public park in Brewster, where the entire 250-strong population of the club went for an end-of-season picnic and awards event. I also attended a staff meeting at the Boys and Girls Club after the summer program ended in order to hear their perspective on what it had been like working with Artie.

The Boys and Girls Club

I saw that there were many commonalities across the two programs. The facility in Brewster, like the one in Wabash, was modern, clean, and attractive. The ratio of staff to youth was similar: at least 25 youth for every staff member. As at Wabash, there were several staff who were quite young, of college age, mixed with more mature staff in their forties. The Brewster club, at least as much as the YRC, catered to a low-income constituency (and a much higher percentage of African Americans), charged a very low fee, and was able to provide free hot lunches, as it, too, was a summer site for the federal nutrition program. Both left their members a great deal of space, without adults hovering over them, and a great deal of autonomy over how they spent their time—but with important differences in the structure of social groupings, as we shall see. Each facility had a TV that hardly anyone watched.

The games area at the Brewster club had many of the same options as the club in Wabash, such as pool and Ping-Pong, with the important difference that nothing required coins to operate. The Brewster game room had two computers loaded with a selection of video games. Both facilities had large gyms and multipurpose rooms that were suitable for arts and crafts or other projects and activities. The Brewster facility had one major activity area that the YRC did not—an upstairs suite of two small, adjoining classrooms, one of which was stocked with state-of-the-art computers, loaded with games as well as learning software. The adjacent room contained tables, chairs, and a blackboard. They called this combined area, which was supervised by one person stationed in either room, their computer and learning lab.[3]

With so many similarities in the ambiance, the demographics of the members, and the activity choices, I was interested to explore what differences between the YRC in Wabash and the Boys and Girls Club in Brewster might justify the inconvenience of the daily drive Artie's family made in both directions. I was able to confirm that all three of the elements that his parents said they were seeking were in fact available for Artie to a greater degree in the summer program he attended in Brewster than they would have been at the YRC.

National Affiliation

Charlotte emphasized that with affiliation with a national organization came the message to all staff that "they have a name, they have a mission, they have standards they have to pay some attention to, they are held accountable." The meaningfulness of the affiliation with national Boys and Girls Clubs of America was borne out during the staff meeting I attended. The assistant operations manager (second in charge of the program) brought up what he called the youth development strategy of their national organization. He said there were three foundations or values to bear in mind, and several of the staff present assisted in recalling and stating what these were: *belonging*, *competence*, and *youthfulness*. They brought this up specifically in connection with the question of whether any name-calling or teasing had taken place during Artie's participation. It appeared that there had been a minimal amount, but they had quickly made it clear that it was inappropriate, that Artie was a member like any other. They emphasized the value of belonging.

When another club member had a question about why Artie acted or spoke the way he did (or repeated things several times), the staff said they would explain that "he has a disability, and we would appreciate if you would look over that, and treat him as a normal person."

During my observations, Artie was sometimes very engaged with other youth and other times conspicuously disengaged (e.g., nodding off to sleep with his head on a table while children around him played a game of hangman). There were times when he was marginalized, but at no time was he stigmatized or excluded.

Artie had at least one good friend who labeled himself as such in a conversation with me at the park. After an organized baseball game ended, this boy continued playing with him informally. At a crowded lunch table, the same boy got other boys to move over and make a space for Artie.

As a group waited in the corridor for their turn in the computer lab, Artie and another boy "slapped five." Then I overheard an exchange that seemed to evidence how fully Artie—obvious developmental differences and all—was accepted by other club members. A boy who had watched him slapping five turned to his companion and said, quietly, "I wish I had a friend like him!" The first boy responded, "I *have* a friend like him." I wasn't sure how exactly to interpret his comment; perhaps he knew someone else with Down Syndrome or another type of special need. What was unmistakable was that both viewed Artie as someone who belonged there and as someone whose presence in the club was desirable.

Charlotte had made the point that the YRC staff were not trained as youth workers, and this was consistent with what I learned from Greg about the way he selected staff at the YRC and the lack of formal staff development activities. I learned that, in contrast, the Boys and Girls Club in Brewster had several trainings per year for their staff, including one every spring that they planned specifically to prepare for their summer program. Because they knew well in advance that Artie would be enrolled, they invited a special educator to conduct a presentation at their spring training. Its focus was not on programming for Artie or other youth with special needs but more on understanding the personal experiences of families that had members with disabilities. At the Boys and Girls Club staff meeting I attended, all felt it had set a good tone for their experience with Artie.

Structure of Social Groupings

Unlike the YRC, where any child could go to any part of the building at any time, the Brewster club subdivided youth by age and required each age group to stay together all day and rotate through four different activity areas (gym, games, multipurpose room, computer and learning lab). The age groups were: 6 to 8, 9 to 10, 11 to 12, and 13 and up.

In the eyes of Artie's father and stepmother, this social structuring accomplished two different and equally important purposes. First, it ensured that their children wouldn't have what they described as "eight hours of hangout time." The requirement that members move around to various areas and experience a balance of athletic, arts-and-crafts, and intellectual challenges appealed to them in regard to all three children, but especially Artie. I saw Artie participate successfully in the games area and the computer lab. The physical education director told me he did fine with the gym activities as well, especially when they played baseball. It did seem, as his parents hoped, that the social structure of the day enabled him to enjoy a balanced and diverse experience. (Left to his own, it looked like he might have chosen Nintendo the entire day.)

There was a second reason why the defined social groupings of the Brewster club appealed to Artie's parents. They worried about the younger siblings, especially Artie's 13-year-old brother, Curt, taking too much of a care taking role for Artie. Although both boys qualified for the 13-and-up group, Artie was assigned, at their request, to the 11 to 12 age group. That way, Curt could be freed to pursue his own friendships and activities without taking on the burden of being spokesperson or guide for Artie.

During an all-day field trip to a public park, there was some breakdown in the structuring of social groupings, and I saw Curt take on the role that worried his father and stepmother. The following is an excerpt from my field notes:

Soon they switch from softball to kickball, not clear how this decision was made. I see the offense and defense switch sides a couple times, but Artie stays off field, by the fence, although he moves closer to those in line when teams are lining up to bat.

Curt has been taking the field and standing in the batting order with one of the teams. I see him get into a tussle with a kid who swipes his baseball cap.

I observed Curt trying to make sure Artie got a turn to bat. Because no staff were organizing the teams . . . the kids formed a line when they came in on offense for a new inning, first come, first served, so you had to move aggressively to kick early in the inning. So Curt pushes Artie forward, saying "Artie hasn't kicked yet." Nobody stopped him from moving him up the line. Still, the third out was made before Artie got to kick.

Finally . . . I see that Artie begins taking a turn in the field, in right field near the edge of the field. He gets verbally into the game now too, yelling out when a fly ball is hit to a teammate: "Catch it." He claps when the player does catch it.

Next offensive chance, Curt is even more aggressive, clapping a hand on Artie's back, gets him in position to be the on-deck kicker when the first one goes up. Artie kicks with confidence, punching a drive in the air to the shortstop, who drops it, allowing him to run safely. Curt runs right along the first base line with him, then turns back.

Curt's role in this sequence of events seemed to be exactly the one his parents were trying to help him avoid, by having him assigned to a separate social group from Artie. It appeared to me that while he invested energy in helping to make sure his brother could participate fully, he was oblivious to the effect it had on his own peer relations. As evidenced by the tussle over the cap referred to in the field notes, those relationships were not uniformly positive. His zealousness in providing moral and physical support to his brother was not likely to improve them.

Curt and Artie's parents and the staff of the Boys and Girls Club had also told me that Artie had a problem limiting food intake. ("He will eat until he's sick," was what his father told me.) During a picnic lunch at the park, I saw Curt take on the caretaker role in respect to Artie's eating as well. I assumed he was just being friendly when he encouraged Artie to sit by him, but Artie—who rejected Curt's overtures and accepted an offer to sit with his other friend—no doubt had a shrewder insight into the family dynamics. Once he shook loose of Curt, he managed to get three hot dogs and an extra bottle of juice. This required full use of his verbal skills and a certain amount of charm. Later, Curt caught up with him. He instructed Artie to get rid of two of the six

cookies he had taken for dessert. Artie complied, silently but unenthu-
siastically, with his younger brother's request.

Style of Supervision

The ratio of staff to youth was stretched at least as thin at the Boys
and Girls Club in Brewster as it was at the YRC in Wabash, so in neither
place could parents expect a child to receive a great deal of individual
supervision. In both places, staff tended to roam and watch for trouble
spots, and expected members to fend for themselves most of the time.

I timed Artie playing Nintendo in the game area at the Brewster club
for 28 minutes, although I learned later there was a rule that you could
only play for 10 minutes if others were waiting—which there were. A
staff member walking through the area eventually yelled to him from
across the room that it was time to switch. (Artie got up right away and
went to one of the pool tables.) In this instance, the laid-back style of
supervision seemed to have been a benefit rather than a problem. The
other children who were sitting with him and rooting him on may have
known that Artie had used up his allotted time, but they seemed to be
drawn to his rapturous aura as he punched the control keys. "Yes! Yes!"
he would say, his voice competing with the synthesized calliope sounds
emanating from the monitor. "I got 'im!" One hand would periodically
reach to the sky, a fist clenched in triumph. "Come on!" "Awesome!"
Sometimes one of the peers watching would give him some advice or
make a comment. But when one girl tried to take over the controls mo-
mentarily, saying, "Artie! Artie! Give it here!" he firmly resisted.

Neither the style of supervision nor the ratio of staff, then, ensured
that a boy like Artie would get the more intensive level of supervision
that his parents told me they were seeking. However, because of the
group structure and the rotation through different areas, there at least
had to be someone paying attention to Artie periodically—if only when
it was time to line up and move to the next area. This was more frequent
attention than he may have gotten in a facility where there was nothing
but unstructured time.

Also, the computer/learning lab was structured more like a classroom, with children working on a combination of individual and group
activities under the more direct supervision of a staff member. That was
an area, therefore, where Artie received more personalized supervision
to accommodate his cognitive differences. I saw the computer/learn-
ing lab teacher, a senior in college, gave him some simple math problems. Another time, she asked him to practice writing his name and

address, while other members wrote stories or poems for a writing contest. She told me this was the sort of assignment she had improvised for him all summer. He sat and worked contentedly at the same table with everyone else in the group. They had different assignments from him, but he was working in proximity and looked like part of their group.

The lunchroom was another place where the staff told me they had learned to modify the rules for him. Ordinarily, they allowed children to eat until they were no longer hungry. But because of the information they received from his family, they limited Artie to first and second helpings only. They also commented on how neatly he handled the chore of straightening up the lunchroom when his age group was finished eating. "He does a better job than some of the staff in folding up the tablecloths," was the way one of them put it.

They acknowledged just one other aspect of his behavior that had required some supervisory attention beyond what was customary. This was his tendency to try to hold or caress either female club members or female staff. His attempts at touching were not blatantly sexual; rather, he would start rubbing an arm or put his arm around a shoulder and say "You my girl." The staff learned from his family that they were setting strict limits on these behaviors at home (with his stepsisters, especially), and they tried to do the same at the club.

Two Programs More Alike Than Different

Artie's family felt confident that the one program would provide him with the support he needed, while they dismissed the other as unworthy of consideration. After spending time in both environments, and becoming familiar with the way they operated, I concluded that the parents were responding more to subtle differences in impressions they received than to any truly dramatic differences in the level of inclusiveness or the overall quality of the programming of the two institutions. The Boys and Girls Club in Brewster and the YRC in Wabash had more similarities than dissimilarities in the experiences they made available and in the ways they supervised and responded to youth members. Several of the dissimilarities we have probed in depth, and I do not mean to dismiss them as trivial. But I do mean to assert that the YRC or any similar program could have earned the trust of a family like Artie's and provided him with an enjoyable summer with just a few extra efforts to get to know his needs and to allay the family's fears and doubts. The first thing the staff at the YRC would have had to do differently was to contact the family after Artie and his stepsister had come to the center and had an unhappy experience the previous summer. I believe the fact that there was no follow-up on that situation was as important to the family, when it came time to make the decision the following year, as any of the positive features of the Boys and Girls Clubs that they articulated to me.

The club in Brewster had not been particularly primed to make Artie's experience a successful one when Artie's father first paid them a visit. At the staff meeting I attended, the operations manager admitted what had been in the back of his mind after the father had made the arrangements to enroll his son. "I figured we'd have to give him a week and then tell his daddy to come get him."

But from the time Artie actually walked in the door, they treated him as if he belonged. Artie acted as if he belonged. And the idea of putting him out of the club never made it to first base.

HOW COULD THE YOUTH RECREATION CENTER BECOME A MORE INCLUSIVE ENVIRONMENT?

Greg was not aware of the unpleasant experience that Artie had when he came to the center the previous summer. (This could be viewed as a by-product of the management style he preferred. Without staff meetings or other formal mechanisms for sharing information or working on staff development, it was unlikely that staff would go out of their way to inform him about an awkward situation such as had arisen with Artie and his stepsister.) But he asserted his belief that the YRC should extend a welcoming hand to any child, with or without disabilities. His main response to the question of what more could be done to make this a reality for all children was to mention how he handled it when a child who was new or shy arrived on the scene. "I find one or two kids and ask them to play with him the first day or two. . . . Just the other day, there was a new boy here who had no one to play with, so I asked a girl to shoot pool with him . . . After that experience, I'm sure he'll be back and feeling a lot less shy."

I shared with Greg some of my observations of the Boys and Girls Club in Brewster and asked him if he could understand why the family, in this case, decided the other environment offered more of what their son needed. Greg acknowledged that having more staff-initiated, structured activities could be a good thing for the YRC. It was something he had thought about over the three years of their operation—not in connection with serving youth with special needs, but as a way of improving the overall strength of the program. He stated that they had moved slowly in that direction. Beginning with a holiday craft event they held last year, they had begun to discover that their members enjoyed doing arts and crafts.

They had no resources to bring in a specialist for this, so the way he described it, either Greg or one of his assistants, once in a while, found an activity in a resource book, got the materials, and set it up in the multipurpose room. He noted that any time they listed arts and crafts on the monthly calendar of activities, their total attendance numbers increased, with an especially big boost in the number of girls. He found that other planned, structured activities, such as bingo, volleyball, and roller-skating, also increased total attendance and were likely to draw equally well among girls and boys (unlike the typical daily club activities, which he acknowledged drew more boys than girls). During one of my observations, I heard several girls ask him, "When are you going to set up the volleyball again?"

Greg agreed that offering more structured, staff-initiated options would be a positive direction that could make the YRC a better place for some of the children who did not currently attend. He could understand that some families of children with special needs might worry about their children feeling left out of basketball or other more free flowing activities and that having more planned and staff-led activities might make it more appealing to them.

But on one point, Greg was adamant. He felt that even if he increased the availability of staff-led activities, they had to be entirely optional. The idea of assigning children to groups or requiring them to rotate in and out of areas did not appeal to him at all. "They go by the clock all day long in school," he said. "They need some creative time when nobody is telling them what they have to do."

When I commented on the extraordinary amount of time some of the youth played basketball to the exclusion of any other activity, he was unfazed. "And that's fine," he said, "if that's what they need to do. . . . I'm 53, and I'm still playing basketball."

Broadening the Range of Activities

Why did more youth (and more girls, especially) attend when they converted the gym to use for roller-skating or volleyball, or when they set up bingo or arts-and-craft activities? Was it because the members had a range of interests and abilities that was wider than what was reflected in the more commonly available activities? Was it because members were hungry for closer contact with an adult (or even a high school–aged leader), contact they could get more easily in a structured activity? I would answer these questions in the affirmative.

A number of members presented repeated behavior problems, got put on time-out, and were threatened with suspension. (Actual suspensions, for periods of days up to months, were rare, but not unheard of.) Eventually, some of them had improved their behavior, while others had stopped coming to the YRC. No doubt, some of these repeat offenders were youth with learning problems. Did they carry on in a socially inappropriate manner in part because they were unable to compete successfully with peers in the rather narrow range of activities that were normally available?

Billy Walls had been a regular user of the center but told me he had become bored and stopped going much—even though he still cited basketball as his main leisure-time activity. His family's lack of resources (they lived in a low-income housing complex) meant the YRC was his only real option for recreational activities, besides playing outdoors. He was 12 years old, had been diagnosed with ADHD, for which he was on Ritalin, and was in special education for his learning disabilities. His mother and stepfather were preoccupied much of the time, dealing with his younger brother who had severe disabilities as a result of a playground accident three years earlier, as discussed in an earlier chapter. They were a family under great duress. It seemed possible that expressing boredom or disenchantment were Billy's coping strategies for a difficult life rather than a well considered reflection on his experience at the YRC. Still, it reinforced a growing hunch I had that nearly everyone—even some of the center's most ardent, basketball-loving patrons—would respond well to the introduction of additional activities that would allow for some changes of pace.

A Welcome for Every Child?

Among the assistants that Greg hired to supervise part-time at the YRC was Bill, a 25-year-old former high school athlete who used a wheelchair. (The origins of his disability were described in an earlier chapter.) In order to teach members of the YRC that a wheelchair was not something to be frightened of (he explained to me), he would sometimes sit on the carpet and let them try wheeling around in his chair.

I commented to Greg that having a staff member who used a wheelchair was sure to make any child who used a wheelchair feel that he or she was entering a receptive setting. He responded that he hoped that was true. He went on to tell me he had been thinking about what to do if a child who used a wheelchair joined the center. He had an idea to get someone to design a lower countertop by the front desk so that the child could sign in while sitting in the wheelchair without having to ask someone else to do it for him.

This statement showed that Greg had thought about the importance of making each child feel welcome, from the moment he or she walked—or wheeled—through the front door. But the statement also left out a great deal. Once he or she signed in, where was Greg expecting the youngster to play? The games area and the music room were not accessible. The basketball gym could have appealed to a wheelchair user who was athletically inclined, provided the staff helped to integrate him or her into the ongoing activities. A creative approach might have involved scheduling times for wheelchair basketball, with 8 or 10 extra wheelchairs obtained for ambulatory hoopsters who did not ordinarily need them. But I saw no evidence that Greg had considered such future possibilities. As the center and its activities were currently configured, it was hard to imagine why a child who used a wheelchair would favor it as a place to spend free time. And even for children who had no physical mobility issues, the range of activities was too narrow to expect children with many kinds of special needs to have fun and make friends there.

Becoming a more inclusive environment would definitely require taking a more proactive approach. The challenges that a young man like Artie presented (e.g., overeating, sexually oriented touching) could be minimized and viewed as minor when there was proper planning and training, as there was at the club he attended in Brewster. But in the absence of training and planning, the same behaviors could have become worse and blown up into a major problem.

In Greg's mind, every youth was welcome and that was an important beginning, a commitment to the goal of inclusion. However, the youth of Wabash with more obvious mental, sensory, or physical disabilities were not using the center. The printed information that was disseminated from the YRC on a regular basis to the broader community never made specific reference to children with disabilities. The hiring and training of staff did not prepare them to take any extra measures when a young man like Artie showed up on the premises. The center, in its few years of operation under the administration of the WPRD, had been successful in offering a recreational alternative to impressive numbers of youth from low-income backgrounds, especially to athletically oriented boys. So far, no one had considered what it would take to make the YRC a more inviting environment for a broader audience that included children with disabilities. There was a vague commitment to the goal of inclusion, but no appreciation for the process that would be required to get there.

On My Honor, I Will Try

"When I was in Girl Scouts, there were no kids like Erica. And I just didn't know if she could be part of it." It was 9:30 A.M., and Katrina, Erica's mother, had put nine-year-old Erica on the school bus, taken her three-year-old to the church-operated preschool, and fed her one-year-old son and put him down for a nap. Finishing a phone call as she invited me to sit in the living room for our scheduled interview, she apologized unnecessarily for her casual attire (shorts and a T-shirt) on an exceptionally warm spring morning.

Mother of a nine-year-old and only 26 years old herself, simple arithmetic told me she was still a high school kid at the time of her pregnancy with Erica. Not immune to stereotypes about teenaged moms, I at first assumed when she told me she was a nurse that she was using the term loosely and meant something like a home health aide—a position that would not have required extensive schooling and rigorous examinations. But my assumption was wrong: She was in fact a registered nurse, having gone back to school when she was 19 and Erica was two years old. Her explanation for what motivated her to get the degree? "To tell you the truth," she said, "I wanted to know what they were saying about my child . . . the nurses and the physician would always be yapping back and forth, all at once." She credited her husband (and father of the three children), a laborer, for supporting her emotionally and financially and in getting her through the nursing program.

Erica was six months old when the parents got the diagnosis of cerebral palsy. "She was making no attempt to sit up, she was tired, there was not a lot of movement." Soon after, the doctors found evidence of heart murmurs (unrelated to the cerebral palsy), which were sapping her energy. "She kind of had a double whammy." Heart surgery—on her first birthday—relieved her energy problem. Since then, she'd been an energetic child, but she had motor problems and also severe delays in speech and communication.

Her walk is what we call a kind of soldier walk, very stiff, like Russian soldiers . . . She plops down when she goes to sit. She can get in and out of the bathtub, but we worry about it. I'm afraid the way she plops down, she'll conk her head and knock herself out.

She falls a lot. She can walk without falling but she's looking around and way ahead and she may not notice something right in front of her. . . . Erica does not know safety. She knows hot and cold, not to touch the stove, but like, she doesn't know not to run in the street. She thinks people will stop, I guess because I've always made sure they did, probably 'cause I've been overprotective.

Her communication is limited. She speaks maybe 10 words. We've tried to teach her sign language. She can do basic signs like "eat," "more," "baby," "drink," "hungry," "please." For "bathroom," she grabs herself; the sign for bathroom is hard for her to get her fingers in position.

NATIONAL ORGANIZATIONS ESPOUSE NEW APPROACHES

According to the Carnegie Council on Adolescent Development (1992), there were at the outset of the 1990s roughly 17,000 organizations offering community-based youth programs in the United States, of which 400 were national in scope. The 15 largest national youth development agencies alone, among which were YMCA, YWCA, Boy Scouts of America, Girl Scouts of the USA, Boys and Girls Clubs of America, Girls Incorporated, Camp Fire Boys and Girls, 4-H, and several others, collectively brushed the lives of 30 million young people per year (National Collaboration for Youth 1990). These organizations dotted the landscapes of our country's smallest towns and largest cities and seemed to offer arenas where young people with special needs might (if they were welcomed) find avenues for friendship, the development of skills, self-expression, and having fun in a group setting. Indeed, some of these organizations had long histories of service to those with disabilities—but, in common with American society as a whole, this was not a history of inclusive practice.

From a Shut-in Society to a Focus on Ability

Prior to the existing national youth programs, there was the Order of the American Boy, headquartered in Detroit, an organization that was founded in 1898 and then dissolved in 1911 after the Boy Scouts came into being.[1] Although it did not consider boys with disabilities as candidates for regular membership, it started a separate association, which was called The American Boy Shut-in Society. An issue of the magazine *The American Boy* from 1901 includes the following discussion. "In our July number we offered to give to any boy who cannot work or play as boys generally do—that is, a boy who is sick or crippled and compelled to remain indoors from morning till night, day after day—one who is likely to be confined to his home for months or years to come, an annual subscription to *The American Boy* free of charge" (1901, 316). The column goes on to give the first and last names of 23 boys who had already responded to the request and continues as follows.

We hope that the reading of *The American Boy* month after month by the little shut-ins will serve to enable them to pass away many hours that otherwise would be wearisome. One letter reads: "I send you a name. The boy in question is a fine, noble hearted boy, very intelligent and cheerful. He will never be able to take a step and has to be carried wherever he goes. To add to his troubles, his parents have lost their entire property within a year."

After quoting excerpts from a number of similar letters, the column concludes with an appeal to readers to "put on their thinking caps and help us to plan some further means of making these boys happy."

The Boy Scouts was founded in 1910 (Boy Scouts of America 1994), and by the 1920s, it had already begun to enable participation by certain members with disabilities. In the 1922 Annual Report, there is a discussion of the possible creation of a new "exempt" class of scouts who are "physically handicapped" and who will be allowed to participate even if they cannot meet the ordinary requirements. "The members of the court of honor feel that the problem of providing for these handicapped scouts is a many-sided one and that some means should be found for encouraging them to do their best without lowering the standard of scouting" (48).

The next year's *Fourteenth Annual Report* (1923) announces that the executive board has taken action "in approving in principle a plan whereby handicapped scouts, that is, crippled boys and other boys not physically capable of passing the second and first class tests, should be awarded special achievement badges and be allowed to earn certain merit badges" (16). To ensure that these honors are not achieved or awarded capriciously, the requirement is that "the handicapped scout shall devise and pass some test within his physical capacity in lieu of the prescribed tests . . . as evidence of his scout spirit and eagerness to develop his ability to the fullest" (48).

These early measures to encourage participation, as in the recreation profession that we discussed in an earlier chapter, did not encompass what became known in later decades as fully inclusive programming. Rather, the idea, in keeping with the thinking of an earlier time, was in most cases to offer boys with special needs their own separate scouting experiences. The 1965 Annual Report trumpets the fact that more than 100 new Scout "units for the handicapped" (71) have been organized that year. The publication announces proudly that this is an all time high.

Reflecting the changing laws and values that were in evidence in the 1970s, the Boy Scouts and numerous other youth serving organizations began to move in a more inclusive direction. *Understanding Cub Scouts with Disabilities* (Boy Scouts of America 1975) was designed to assist volunteer leaders in working with boys with special needs within regular Cub Scout dens that served typically developing peers. During that same period, the national YMCA, with the help of federal funds, initiated a collaborative effort called Project May (Mainstreaming Activities for Youth) that involved many of the other major youth development agencies and resulted in a series of three manuals (Young Men's Christian Associations of the USA 1980). The Boys Clubs (not yet reorganized at that time to form the Boys and Girls Clubs of America) issued a publication called *Mainstreaming Matters* (Boys Clubs of America 1985). A leader's guide was developed within the 4-H system to promote involvement of youth with disabilities (Cooperative Extension Service of Purdue University n.d.). More recently, the Girl Scouts issued *Focus on Ability/Serving Girls with Special Needs* (Carroll 1990).

Some initiatives were also in evidence at the local level. In Minneapolis and St. Paul, Minnesota, three different public and private agencies collaborated over a two-year period, beginning in 1993, in procuring a grant from a local foundation and introducing a series of measures to make their programs and activities more available and accessible to young people and adults with disabilities. The agencies were the Camp Fire Boys and Girls, the YMCA, and the Park and Recreation Board (Vinland 1995). An example of a change introduced was that a flyer promoting a summer class in golfing for youth from 8 to 16 years old featured a line drawing of a girl sitting in a wheelchair, hitting a golf ball with an oversized club, next to another golfer swinging a normal club from the conventional standing position.

The newsletter of the Girl Scouts of the USA (1994, May, 1) reported that more than 47,000 girls with disabilities were members of regular troops in 1993, up by more than 5,000 from the year before. They noted that this number came to only about 1 in 33 of all girls with disabilities, and only 1.8 percent of all Girl Scouts, making them the "most underrepresented group in our present membership." Nevertheless, that was a long way up the road (and nearly a century in time) from the days when children with disabilities had to be thankful to be members of a Shut-in Society, with their closest connection to a youth program being a subscription to a magazine.

TO JOIN THE GIRL SCOUTS: NOT A SIMPLE DECISION

Katrina had been a Girl Scout herself. But when I met the family, her daughter Erica was not among the 47,000 Girl Scouts with identified disabilities, nor was she involved in any other comparable activities. She attended school, joined the family on outings to the swimming pool, and played with her siblings and the next-door neighbors' children. But she was not having the kind of peer-oriented, group experiences common to other kids her age.

Erica attended a special education classroom in the Wabash public schools. (The year her parents moved to their current home from Brewster was the first year students with her level of disability were assigned to classrooms within the local elementary schools.) When the school sent home information inviting parents to sign up their daughters for Girl Scouts, Katrina wrote a note to the aide that worked with Erica during the school day to ask if she thought they would take her. The aide called and said she "had heard they had some handicapped kids." But at the time, Katrina was busy with her newborn son, and her inquiry went no further.

In truth, the thought of signing up Erica for the Girl Scouts led directly in Katrina's mind to a host of other questions that she had not yet resolved for herself. These related to how much protection and support

Erica needed—not only at her current age but even into the rather distant future.

I don't want someone to make fun of her. . . . My husband has a 10-year-old brother; he's not around much but when he is around her, he will make fun of her. She flaps her arms at times, and he'll flap his arms to make fun of her.

She loves to do things away from us, not just with the three kids and us. I know it would be good for her to be with other kids . . . but you hear so much about camp counselors abusing children. I don't know if I could control myself if something like that happened. My husband says, think about when we get older, we're not going to be with her everywhere she goes. But I can't let myself think about that.

When my husband was younger, he was kind of an overseer for a group home for kids from about age 18 to 25. And he has said, this is probably the kind of place Erica will be in some day. But they had people coming in and talking about sex. I mean actually telling them how to do it. . . . I just don't see her as cognitively being able to deal with that kind of information. . . . There was one girl in this group home that got pregnant. And she *wanted* to get pregnant. I just don't know if I can ever accept that! . . . Erica was with me at the doctor's just recently, and he said she was at the low end of normal for starting her period!

When I had a chance to reflect on the substance of this interview, it struck me as unlikely that moms of other eight-or nine-year-olds, girls without disabilities—in Wabash or anywhere else—were bringing such a complex web of present and future concerns to what many must consider a simple decision about whether to sign up a child for a scout troop. But at least for this one parent of a child with special needs, a decision to put her in Girl Scouts was charged with emotion. It raised concerns in her mind about how other children would respond, and fears about adult leaders who might be irresponsible, insensitive to her individual needs, or worse. These worries in turn were related to Katrina's anxieties about what level of functioning, competence, and independence her daughter would attain in the future, as far as 10 to 15 years down the road.

I did not attempt to help Katrina resolve these larger issues. However, because I had already met with some paid and volunteer leaders of the local Girl Scouts, I was able to reassure her on at least one point. If you sign Erica up for Girl Scouts, I told her, she does not have to attend without you. All parents, I knew, were welcome to attend the troop meetings. I also asked her what steps, if any, a group like the Girl Scouts could take to make her feel comfortable in signing up her daughter.

Haltingly, she responded, "If I was sure they would take her and treat her like the other kids, and if I have the option to drop in any time, and stand back and watch, and I know they're fair . . . "

AN IN-DEPTH LOOK AT THE BROWNIE TROOP THAT ERICA JOINED

The following fall, Katrina did sign Erica up for Girl Scouts. She was assigned not to a Junior Girl Scout troop, for which she was eligible by her age, but for Brownies. (This was a decision arrived at jointly, between parent, troop leader, and "troop consultant," a position filled by a volunteer who helped organize all the troops in a single community. If a parent of a child with disabilities preferred that the girl remain with her chronological peers, they would have respected that preference.)

The Brownie troop to which Erica was assigned already included one other girl with special needs among its 10 members and had as its leader Francine, a special education teacher with 18 years of experience in the Wabash public schools. LaToya turned 10 during the year of the study and therefore was also old enough to be a Junior Girl Scout, but her mother, like Erica's, believed that she would benefit more from being with the younger girls in Brownies.

LaToya was African American and small-framed, but there was no longer any evidence of the near-starvation weight of 12 pounds that she tallied at the age of two and one-half years, when Martha and her husband had adopted her. She wore wire rim glasses, and on the few occasions I saw her, she seemed to keep her head angled to her left most of the time, while sitting in her wheelchair.

At school, LaToya was in a classroom with just two to three other special education students with multiple and severe disabilities. (She was assigned to music and recess with typically developing peers.) Although she still spent most of her day in a segregated classroom, her mother, Martha, was jubilant about the fact that she no longer had to put her on a bus all the way to Brewster for school. She was just completing her first year of this new arrangement when I met them. Martha, like Katrina, was also a nurse by training, but with LaToya plus five other children still at home, was not currently employed in her profession. She worked part-time making floral arrangements and pointedly informed me that her nursing skills were very much in use—with four children with cerebral palsy (two she denoted as severe), three of whom had seizure disorders, and two of whom had multiple medical challenges.

LaToya needed someone else to push her wheelchair from place to place, due to lack of upper body strength. For expressing her thoughts and requests, she used an augmentative communication device called a Liberator. The Liberator was programmed to play prerecorded words or phrases. When LaToya activated the device with a movement of her head (because she had limited use of her arms and hands), a series of words or phrases were pronounced at the level of a whisper, so that she could hear them. (This, her mother explained to me, was called auditory prompting.) Once she found the phrase or expression she wanted, she could press an extra time on the head switch to have the Liberator speak it again, louder, once or several times, for the benefit of those with whom she was communicating.

At one troop meeting, we were making napkin rings by coloring little Pilgrim faces and then cutting and gluing them onto one-inch segments of paper towel rolls. LaToya found on her Liberator what must have been the phrase most proximate in content: "I like to play with paper dolls!" She played this comment at least seven or eight times.

One unusually long expression that Martha had programmed into LaToya's Liberator, after she joined the Brownies, was the Girl Scout Promise:

> On my honor, I will try:
> To serve God and my country,
> To help people at all times,
> And to live by the Girl Scout Law.

Martha was proud of the fact that LaToya was able to learn to retrieve and play back the Promise at appropriate times. (All the phrases programmed into the Liberator were categorized by themes; each theme was represented by one of 32 icons, which were visible in four rows of eight, under Plexiglas, on the tray attached in front of her wheelchair. To retrieve a particular phrase meant accessing the correct theme first and then auditory scanning to the desired expression—a very challenging process.)

Besides her need for special supports in the areas of communication and mobility, LaToya also took her nourishment through a tube and wore glasses on account of visual impairment. Her lack of manual dexterity meant that she needed someone to give her hand-over-hand assistance with typical Brownie activities, for instance, arts-and-crafts tasks, such as drawing and cutting. Martha regarded her daughter as very so-

cial and having a strong personality, in spite of the barriers to typical social interactions.

She's opinionated. She doesn't like math. The teacher goes crazy because of
that. So we've got a rule, like any other kid, that she does not watch the Flint-
stones if she hasn't done her math. She likes to be around other people; she's a
very social child. This is one of the reasons I pursued her getting into Girl
Scouts with kids that were age-appropriate and getting into a Sunday school
class with kids at church.

The Setting and the Other Troop Members

Martha may not have known what she was going to miss when she
dispatched her husband to the troop meeting with LaToya on the eve of
Valentine's Day. LaToya's attendance at meetings had been inconsistent. For the benefit of a one-hour social experience with typically developing peers, Martha had to take herself, LaToya, the wheelchair, and
the Liberator onto the van, drive to the Church of Christ, make two
trips from the parking lot to bring LaToya and her paraphernalia inside,
then do it all in reverse when the meeting ended. As it happened, La-
Toya also had physical therapy the same afternoon, which was very
draining. Each Thursday at supper time, Martha had to decide if La-
Toya (and mom too) had enough energy left to make the trip to the
Brownie meeting worthwhile.

January snowstorms had caused two regularly scheduled meetings
to be canceled. The upshot was that LaToya hadn't made it to a meeting since before the Christmas holidays.

As troop members, mostly second-graders, arrived, they stepped
jauntily into a huge, mostly undecorated, multipurpose room, with an
outside wall made of painted cinderblocks, green curtains on two large
windows, and a ceiling two-stories high made of curved wooden
beams. There were numerous folding tables and chairs set out and even
more folded and stacked out of the way; the room could have seated
150 people with no problem if they were all set up. You could guess the
uses to which this Fellowship Hall was put at other times by the stage
and upright piano down to the left as you entered from the side and a
spacious kitchen at the opposite end.

Parents walked their kids inside the foyer of the church, which separated the outside door from the meeting room, proceeding just far
enough to make sure the leaders were there to receive them, and then
flashed a quick good-bye. Each girl removed her winter coat as she en-

tered the room. Some were more fastidious than others as they piled them onto a table near the entrance.

The hall was looking and sounding unusually festive. A portable stereo was booming contemporary music. On one table dozens of little valentines spilled out, waiting for children to address them to one another. On another table appeared other kinds of arts-and-crafts materials, and hats made out of folded newspaper. These preparations had been made by Francine and Tammy, the volunteer leader and assistant leader, who had arrived first along with Francine's two daughters, Grace and Annie. Annie was one of the Brownies, and all the girls knew Grace, her 16-year-old sister, very well by now. She had shared the leadership of the troop all year long, thereby fulfilling one of her requirements, as a Senior Girl Scout, for the Gold award.

This was Francine's second year as a troop leader. Tammy worked in the same classroom with her as a paraprofessional and had been recruited by Francine this past fall as a volunteer, although Tammy's two children were not yet old enough to be scouts. Martha's youngest child was in Francine's special education classroom, and Tammy was his aide. Thus, Martha knew the two leaders quite well and was on very friendly terms with them. In fact, on more than one occasion, when LaToya was unable to attend Brownies, Martha came on her own, anyway, and helped out.

With their coats off, you could see that the girls were impressively diverse in their clothing, shapes, sizes, and ethnic and racial identities, as well as abilities and disabilities. Leaders in several Girl Scout troops I visited (and Boy Scout leaders too) told me that they could not require children to wear uniforms, even though that might contribute to the sense of group identity, because too many of the families found the cost prohibitive. On this particular evening, only Darcy, an African American, wore a Brownie sash over her blouse, combined with the traditional, chocolate brown Brownie skirt. (Darcy was the biological sister of Carlton, whose participation in tee-ball we discussed in an earlier chapter. They were foster children in the home of Steve and Sheila.)

There were skirts or dresses on two of the three Asian American girls, while everyone else wore pants. The third African American girl (after LaToya and Darcy) was dressed in the splashiest outfit of all: a multicolored, nylon sweat suit. One of the four European American girls was slightly taller and far heftier than anyone else, easily carrying double the weight of the smallest girls.

How Erica Presented Herself

Erica and LaToya, with their respective disabilities, added another kind of diversity. Erica's demeanor was friendly, open, smiling. She had curly, close cropped blondish hair and rosy cheeks. Her weight was in proportion to her height; she looked about the right size among a group of seven-year-olds. The first meeting I observed her, I heard one of the other troop members ask her mom how old she was. "Would you believe, she's nine?" Katrina answered. "She's really small, isn't she?"

The stiff "Russian soldier" walk her mom had told me about was noticeable, but what accentuated her developmental differences was not her walk as much as the way she interacted with people. She didn't speak (or was only beginning to use some words and vocalizations), but seemed to use physical touch as her way of getting and keeping the attention of a peer or adult. Over the course of several meetings, I saw her try different approaches, from full frontal hugging to taking a hairband off another girl's head and putting it on her own to strongly taking hold of both hands of another person (adult or child) and pulling on them in one direction or another.

At the end of the first meeting that I observed her, she took hold of one of my hands and the hand of a peer and tried to get us to hug one another. When I demurred and gave a friendly handshake instead, a little storm cloud of unhappiness formed on Erica's face. She actually appeared to tear up, just for a minute. "Erica really likes everybody to hug each other," said Katrina, who was standing nearby.

Erica's gestures were invariably accompanied by smiles and sometimes by sounds. But although her face expressed benevolence, the forcefulness of her physical motions and the strong grip of her fingers sometimes seemed to disclose an underlying frustration or discontent. I had met Erica's grandmother before I met the parents, and she had told me she thought Erica was getting more angry and frustrated due to the lack of a communication outlet. Katrina had acknowledged that she could be aggressive (even though she was gentle and loving most of the time) toward her three-year-old sister and baby brother, especially.

She's very protective over her baby dolls; she loves playing with dolls. . . . If her sister touches one of her dolls that she doesn't want her to, she pinches, bites, pulls her hair, anything to get her to do what she wants. But when she's playing with them, she treats them real nice, holds her baby just like a mom (demonstrates).

She's not aggressive toward her dolls? (I asked.)

No.

To you?

Not really. If she's expected to do something, because we do expect her to do certain things, she will be disciplined for that, and if she doesn't and she yells, we'll send her to her room, and on her way she spits at you. She may pinch at you. When she was little she would bite us.

My son takes a bottle and she knows that and she wants to shove the bottle in his mouth. If he doesn't want it, she'll push. I know she's not trying to be forceful, she thinks he needs it. . . . . When [three-year-old sister] was a baby, one time we heard her crying and Erica was in there, trying to change her diaper.

The Valentine's Day party had been planned at another troop meeting three weeks earlier. Grace had divided us into two groups, one to generate food plans and one to think of activities, with one girl in each group holding pencil and paper, recording everyone's suggestions. LaToya had missed that meeting, but Tammy and I sat with the group that included Erica.

She did not speak, and only with some effort did we manage to keep her sitting at the table with us during the brief discussion. Her eyes and her attention wandered as the other Brownies wrote down ideas of what to eat and drink. I was seated next to the Brownie making the list for our group and facing Erica across the table, with my hands on the table in front of me. Erica reached across and touched one of my hands. Very deliberately and attentively she gazed at it and probed my closed fist with one finger the way a baby six months to a year old might do. When I squeezed and unsqueezed my fist around the finger she had inserted there, she got a bubbly look on her face. But when one of the other girls mentioned "popcorn," all of a sudden, it recaptured Erica's interest. Francine, who had been watching from a distance, walked over and asked her, "Erica, you want to have popcorn at the party? Everybody, raise your hand if you want popcorn." The other girls raised their hands, and so did Erica.

How LaToya Presented Herself

Martha and LaToya had first been exposed to some of the local Girl Scout leaders through the Focus on Ability activities, which are described later in this chapter. Martha had accepted an invitation on two different occasions to bring LaToya to these workshops as a guest speaker, to explain to the troop members about some of the toys and equipment LaToya had, and about her individual needs. Rosemary, who had put me in touch with Martha, was also the one who had invited her to the Focus on Ability event. Subsequently, Martha called her to see about getting LaToya into the Girl Scouts as an active member and was pleasantly surprised at how easy it was.

The leaders were very welcoming, and so were the girls. Martha commented especially on two Asian American girls who seemed extremely friendly to LaToya. "If one of them sees that she's operating her Liberator, they'll say, 'LaToya's getting ready to talk—everybody be quiet!'"

There were no meetings during the summer. When the troop began to meet again in the fall, LaToya was still recovering from surgery she had in July and was not ready to go out to the evening meetings. As an alternative, Martha invited the troop to meet at her home. They held two meetings there, and during these meetings, the girls had a chance to play with some of LaToya's adapted toys (some had switches that set off movement, lights, or noises) and learn more about her equipment and her ways of coping with her disabilities. For example, Martha demonstrated how she lowered LaToya into and raised her out of her bathtub using a lift. Each girl (except for one who didn't want to) climbed onto the lift, fully clothed, and tried it out for herself.

The other troop members, then, were still getting to know LaToya. Surrounded by paraphernalia, attended by a parent at all times, and unable to be present with consistency, she was made fully welcome but remained a bit of a mystery to the other girls, as far as I could tell. They showed curiosity, interest, kindness. But up until the evening of the Valentine's Day party, none of them approached her in the same carefree way they approached one another.

Hearts and Laughter at a Valentine's Day Party

The meetings at Martha's house were the first ones that Erica attended. They also turned out to be the only ones, prior to the Valentine's Day party, at which both Erica and LaToya had been present together. Erica must have remembered being with LaToya at her house four months earlier: From the moment her dad wheeled her into the Fellowship Hall, Erica's behavior toward her long-absent peer, in contrast to that of all the other girls, was effusive and aggressively friendly. Lacking the oral language and the social inhibitions of the other troop members, and using physical touch as her way of initiating social interactions, Erica was unrelenting and irrepressible in her overtures toward LaToya. LaToya responded to virtually everything Erica did with joy and animation. She lit up with smiles and laughter that I had not previously witnessed. I wrote the following in my field notes:

What was really obvious and made the evening so special was that Erica clearly was very excited to see LaToya and could barely leave her alone all evening (and dad was very cool with this). And LaToya, in turn, clearly enjoyed Erica's attention. Erica would push her face right up to her. She had to be limited at times when she would try to undo the velcro that holds a bicycle-type horn to her tray and when she tried to push the icons under the Plexiglass on LaToya's Liberator, too. Once she even tried to shake her wheelchair. LaToya's dad put her off in a very relaxed way, but what was obvious was that LaToya really liked having her intense attention. Several different times, Erica got her laughing and smiling. Erica said "tickle tickle tickle" at least once, and more than once, she used her fingers to tickle her.

Grace organized the girls into three groups: pizza baking (tomato sauce, grated cheese, and pepperoni on English muffins), addressing valentines to other troop members (Tammy taped a list of all the names, printed large, on the wall), and decorating newspaper hats. Grace asked me to coordinate the hat decorating at one table; her mom was doing the pizza in the kitchen, and Tammy did the valentines. Later, we blew up balloons, lots of pink, white, and red ones, enough for everybody to take two home. The last few minutes was snack time: eating the miniature pizzas and drinking soft drinks. The balloons, a two-liter bottle of cola, and a few other contributions came from the girls, in keeping with the decisions we made three weeks earlier. Evidently, popcorn did not make the final cut (or perhaps, whoever agreed to bring it did not).

The three groups did not endure as fixed social groupings (girls would finish something and move along, not worrying about where they were supposed to be). At the beginning, however, I did see rare evidence of a typically developing peer showing discomfort with the troop's inclusive character. Grace had divided the girls up by counting them off. By unplanned consequence, her sister, Annie, was grouped with LaToya, Erica, and no other Brownies. They started at my hat-decorating table. As we began our activity, Annie, who was always jovial and energetic but also not one to hold back her opinions, said to no one in particular, something like, "I always get stuck with . . . " and glanced around at the two girls with disabilities. She let her sentence trail off, and then, directly to me, she added, "I'm glad you're here!" I did not hear it as an expression of hostility or nonacceptance toward the two girls but as a kind of plaint: How can I have fun when I'm matched up with two peers with whom it is impossible to have conversations? (Annie was usually the chattiest member of the troop—not an easily earned accolade among girls this age.)

I tried out a couple of different newspaper hats Grace had made on LaToya's head (she didn't seem to mind), until one seemed to fit properly. Her dad said, in a very friendly way, "Oh, it kind of looks like a nurse's hat; LaToya's mother is a nurse." We then placed the hat on her tray, and her dad helped her to lick and stick on paper hearts that Grace had prepared in advance of the meeting.

LaToya was in her wheelchair, and the rest of us were seated on two sides of a long table a few feet away. Erica was much more interested in LaToya than in decorating her own hat, so I encouraged her to come over and help LaToya and her dad with their decorating. Erica flapped her arms in excitement as she stood close to LaToya. (I would see her do this several times during the evening.) She did help a little and then it was hard to convince her to go back to work on her own hat. Grace tried to get her to return to her original seat, which was all the way around the other side of the long table. I suggested Erica could take my seat, which was the closest one to LaToya's wheelchair, a suggestion Grace accepted. We got Erica to do only a little more on her own hat, as she mostly clung—visually, when not physically—to the action at LaToya's tray.

In the kitchen, her dad helped LaToya to spoon tomato sauce onto a pizza. There, too, we were not able to get Erica to do much of the task, as her interest was much more on her companion. When we began to blow up balloons, Erica left LaToya alone for a while and got very interested in the balloons. She acted afraid of them at first, walking far away, standing near the piano, toward the other end of the long room. But she soon got over her apparent fear, bouncing a balloon back and forth with me, knocking it up high, and seeming to learn—after verging on tears the first time it happened—that even when one smacked her in the face, it did not hurt. Other girls helped to blow up balloons and were also sending them around the room, as Erica and I played together.

When it was time for everyone to eat a snack, Tammy sat with La-Toya by the valentine table, holding a crayon, hand-over-hand, helping her address envelopes to the other Brownies and writing her own name on the back. Although LaToya could not eat with the others (because she took her nourishment through a G-tube), I wondered why Tammy didn't bring her over to join the other girls, just to be part of this communal activity now that we were no longer divided into our three separate subgroups.

It was a very relaxed time, after intense engagement in the three activities and the balloons. One group of three girls was comparing the ages of their respective brothers. Others were commenting on the pizza. LaToya's dad took a break to eat a pizza, while Tammy tended to his daughter. In between snacking, three of the girls got up from the table to dance the macarena, a dance that had become particularly popular among all age groups—but especially among school-aged and preadolescent girls, it seemed—at the time. (Grace had put on a tape of the requisite song.)

Francine and Grace, beginning to pick up the remnants of the evening's activities, allowed the girls their own autonomous space to carry on conversations. They tried to get Erica to come to the table and eat her pizza. Tammy tried too, and so did I, but she chose, once again, to hang around by LaToya and Tammy. LaToya continued to appear to be pleased by her attention. Erica never did eat any snack.

I commented to Francine on how much interaction there had been between LaToya and Erica. She, too, had seen some of the touching, tickling, and laughing. "It could be that the two of them can communicate with each other better than we'll ever be able to," she smiled.

Several questions drifted through my mind as I sat next to Erica's empty chair. Was the fact that Erica could relate so well to LaToya (and that LaToya so obviously appreciated her overtures) an argument against inclusive practice, an illustration that "these kinds of kids" would benefit more from segregated programs specifically set up for those with disabilities? Was it bad that the two girls with visible special needs were physically separated from the other eight girls? What signal, if any, did this send to the other girls? How important was it to get Erica to do the "socially appropriate" thing by having her come to eat her snack with the other troop members? Would there have been any real value in wheeling LaToya over to the snack table, even though she wouldn't eat and wouldn't be able to join in the conversations? Meanwhile, the other girls, absorbed in relaxed conversation and pizza, did not seem to be aware that two of their companions were engaged in a different part of the room. Did they even think of Erica and LaToya as having an identity in common with each other and different from the rest of them, an identity that adults conceptualized as "children with disabilities"?

What was unmistakable, in spite of these unresolved questions, was that all the girls were having a great time—those in the snack area and the two with Tammy by the valentines. All of them were part of one Brownie troop. Everybody accepted everyone else as being part of the experience (that even extended to me, the gray-haired guy from Brewster, who jotted down notes once in a while in a pocket-sized spiral notebook). Why would you want to change anything when everyone had achieved such contentment? That too was a question I asked myself later that evening as I typed my field notes back in my own apartment.

AN OVERVIEW OF INCLUSIVE GIRL SCOUTING IN WABASH

LaToya and Erica were not the first or only girls with disabilities to join Girl Scout troops in Wabash. Lindy (profiled in an earlier chapter) had been a Junior Girl Scout until her death the previous year. Seven-year-old Ariana was a member of Francine's Brownie troop at the time I initiated the community case study but had been reassigned to a different troop by the time I started my visits to their meetings. We reviewed her medical history in an earlier chapter: Ariana stopped walking at age 10 months and was eventually diagnosed with Guillain-Barré syndrome. Aside from having to use a wheelchair, she was communicating and functioning very much at or above the level of her ambulatory peers.

During the summer break, Francine and the volunteer Girl Scout consultant for the area decided that half the Brownies from her troop would be assigned to a new troop, in order to keep it from becoming overly large. Ariana was one of those who became part of the new troop, whose meetings I also attended.

Jennifer, age 12, had attended Daisies (for kindergarten-age girls) and Brownies (for ages six to eight), and at the time of the study was active in Junior Girl Scouts, which serves grades 3 through 6, or ages 9 through 12. The troop in which she was active had 15 members and was led by Gretchen, who had been her leader since the beginning, except for one year when she was unavailable for evening activities due to working a second shift in one of the local factories.

Jennifer had light-brown hair of medium length and wore wire-rimmed glasses. I noted more than once in my field notes that her face was both pretty and serene. The latter was not an adjective I had occasion to use in describing other children I observed; in fact, I often made note of girls or boys who appeared stressed, in a hurry, or frazzled. With cheeks that still showed a bit of baby fat, her face also looked younger than many of her peers. I wondered if her deafness—her being somewhat shielded from the noise, the hustle-bustle, and the cultural messages that poured into the ears of inhabitants of the hearing world—had worked to her benefit, promoting her serenity and preserving her younger look. She had worn a cochlear implant for several years now, so she was not quite so fully shielded from the hearing world as she had been in her younger years. In fact, Gretchen quoted a comment Jennifer had made that seemed to support my intuition about her development. After undergoing the surgery for the implant and trying it out for a while, she signed, "I don't like your world. It's too loud."

Too much "talking and talking"

When I interviewed Jennifer, with her 21-year-old sister Laurie as my interpreter, I printed my questions (the ones I could think of ahead of time) in advance on note cards. I handed them across the kitchen table in their home, one at a time, and as Jennifer and Laurie read them, Laurie sometimes embellished with signs. Jennifer was very responsive in the interview, and Laurie told me she thought that writing down the questions made it much easier for her.

As with other interviews I conducted with children, I began with questions that were not directly related to the topic of my inquiry. I wanted to help my respondents to get comfortable with the interview process and to understand that there were no "correct" answers, that their thoughts, opinions, and feelings were important to me. Jennifer responded with enthusiasm to a question I asked about whether she had any best friends. She identified two of them: Both were deaf, and neither of them lived in Wabash. Complicating matters further, she was not in school with either of them this year, because she had transitioned from elementary to junior high school. One friend had made the same transition but to a different junior high. The other was a year behind and was still at the elementary school.

Jennifer had gone to school all her life in Brewster, and these examples highlighted the difficulty of making friends in her own neighborhood and community. Her parents had brought up this subject as well when I interviewed them. They told me that one of her best friends lived about 20 miles from Brewster, which made it 35 to 40 miles away from them and not easy to make social plans together with any frequency.

When I asked Jennifer if it was hard to try to make friends in both Wabash and Brewster, she replied by saying she had to go to school in Brewster "because there's no interpreters here in Wabash." She added that it wasn't hard anymore, because she knew so many people in both places, but "when I was younger, I used to ask myself, 'why am I here in Brewster?'"

Horses and Hikes

Jennifer told me that there was a lot she liked about Girl Scouts, including "making friends," "helping people," and "doing fun things." She became very animated in describing the two times that the troop had worked on a patch related to horses. "The first time I rode a horse, people had to lead the horse around. The second time, I was riding by myself." She had been on some overnights, sleeping both in a tent and in a cabin. She enjoyed it and specifically mentioned swimming and "eating the marshmallows." "You know," Laurie added, to me, "the smores" (the well known Girl Scout combination of graham crackers with chocolate and marshmallows).

Jennifer had never gone camping for a full week along with the rest of the troop members, however. Her mom told me she had never sent her because there would not have been any sign language interpreters available (as far as Patsy could determine).

Jennifer had a very favorable view of her total experience. But was there anything she didn't like? Yes: "talking and talking and talking," she signed. That Jennifer's attention wandered during certain portions of the troop meetings had been readily apparent during my observations. The more they were involved in a hands-on, multisensory activity, such as New Games, braiding each other's hair, or doing a craft project, the more she was engaged and attentive. But there were many discussions geared to making decisions about patches, fund-raising, and social events. During these discussions, I watched her become very obviously disengaged. Several times, I saw her initiate a conversation with her mom or sister, in sign language, accompanied by occasional whispered vocalizations, oblivious to what the troop was discussing. Other times, she took a bathroom break or let her gaze drift to other parts of the room.

Feeling Left Out

Jennifer described the "talking" parts of the meetings as boring. (During our interview, she taught me the American Sign Language sign for "boring"; you pick at your nose with your index finger.) But when I asked her if she felt left out at these times, she responded with a more literal example than I had anticipated.

When I used the phrase, I meant only to convey the sense of being cut off from some of the communication. But she responded by talking of times when the girls broke into pairs or small groups to do activities. "When we get ready to start an activity, all the girls choose someone to do it with, and I end up with whoever is left after that."

This was certainly a poignant observation that went to the heart of the success or failure of inclusion. In the five meetings of her troop that I attended, I had not observed her being the last one left to be chosen for a paired or small group activity. Yet even if this happened only occasionally, its occurrence was seared into her memory.

Her remarks reminded me of a passage from a favorite book of mine, Geoffrey Wolff's personal memoir, *The Duke of Deception* (1979, 119). The author described his efforts at forming friendships after his parents were divorced and he had moved with his mom to a different state. He was eleven years old, nearly the same age as Jennifer. "I had a friend. Ernie lived in a trailer park just off the Tamiami Trail. Our derelict Schwinns brought us together. . . . Ernie was the grungiest kid in class, and it upset my mother that I chose him for my friend. I didn't choose, he didn't choose, we were all that was left after the others chose."

When I asked Jennifer if any of the girls had done something to make her feel more included and not left out, she again invoked the experience of having to pair off for an activity. She described one girl, whose name she did not know, by her hair and glasses. When the group broke up into pairs, she said this girl had chosen to work with her on a couple of occasions. Her capacity to recollect these occasions spoke powerfully of how much they had meant to her.

When I asked Jennifer, "Can you think of any ideas that would make it easier for you to participate in troop meetings," she said no. After a pause, she added, "just to make more friends in Wabash."

Laurie was the second oldest of four children and one of two whose hearing was unimpaired. Both Laurie and their older sister had gone all the way through Girl Scouts, winning the silver and gold awards, the organization's highest honors. Jennifer had told her sisters that she aspired to do the same. Part of the requirement to earn these awards was to work with younger Girl Scouts, as Grace was doing in her mom's Brownie troop. Jennifer had specifically told Laurie she wanted to do that, just the same as her big sisters.

Laurie expressed to me privately, after my interview with Jennifer was finished, that she worried about whether Jennifer would be able to fulfill these ambitions. She recalled that as she entered the Cadettes (which came after Juniors, and would begin the next year for Jennifer), there was even more group discussion than in Juniors. "A lot of gossiping, a lot of sitting around talking about what boys we liked, and other things. Kind of like a counseling session." If Jennifer already felt discontented with the amount of talking in her current troop, Laurie thought she would find the Cadettes even more boring.

Another meaningful part of Laurie's experience as a Senior Girl Scout had been attendance at out-of-state events, including a conference in Savannah, Georgia, birthplace of Juliet Gordon Lowe, the founder of the organization. Could she envision her sister participating in such an event and enjoying it as much as Laurie did? "To tell you the truth, I've never seen a hearing-impaired Girl Scout on those trips. . . . She would need someone to interpret." She definitely did not find viable the idea of having herself or their mom along to interpret, as they did at the weekly meetings. She feared Jennifer might end up dropping out and not achieving her ambition to attain the silver and gold awards.

Modifying Activities

Gretchen stated that because Jennifer was a bright child who could do anything the other girls could do, she did not consider it essential or appropriate to consider each activity with respect to how Jennifer might do it, or whether it needed any adaptation. She felt the only issue was making sure it was communicated to her. My observations were consistent with Gretchen's comments: I saw no examples of program or activity modifications for her benefit. However, leaders of other local troops responded differently to this question.

The patches that the Brownies earn are called Try-Its. Martha told of how she helped the leaders to modify two of these so that LaToya could accomplish the tasks. The first one involved using different senses.

They put their hands in a bag and feel if they can find two objects that are exactly the same. But LaToya couldn't put her hands in a bag, so what we did was put four things on her tray, and then the Senior Girl Scout who was helping to lead the troop would hold up two at a time and ask if they were the same. When they weren't alike, LaToya wouldn't respond, but when they were the same, she would have a big smile on her face. The girl was very impressed. She exclaimed, "she's getting them all right!"

The other Try-It that Martha worked on with her daughter had to do with animals:

They're supposed to go in the woods and look at the habitat. Well, there aren't too many woods that are accessible to a person in a wheel-chair. So, LaToya is into animal movies, like the new Lassie, the Panda story from China, and

Homeward Bound. So, we would use these movies, and pause the video, and ask her questions, like, does this animal live in a tree? And she would answer the questions.

And you had her demonstrate this? I asked.

No, we wrote up a paper. If the girls work on a badge at home, that's what you do. And the leaders said that what LaToya did was more in-depth than the girls who went into the woods to get the patch.

Lucy and Celeste were the leaders of the Brownie troop that formed when Martha's troop was divided. They took Ariana's physical disability into account when they chose activities and sometimes revised their plans to accommodate her. One Try-It they picked out to do during the good weather, early in the fall, was the outdoor sports one. They looked it over carefully to see if there was some way for Ariana to participate, because the requirement in the Brownies manual was to complete four of six activities listed. "But with options like roller-skating around cones and bicycling, there was just no way. We thought of putting her in charge of starting and stopping and timing the others with a stopwatch, but we weren't comfortable with that. So we dropped that one. There ended up not being enough good weather in the fall, so we probably wouldn't have been able to do it anyway."

They spoke of one meeting when they decided it was time to have fun and not worry about completing another Try-It. Using funds they had in their troop treasury from the 20 percent of the proceeds that they kept when their members sold calendars and candy in the fall, they treated the group to supper at the local McDonald's, which had a play space. (They had called up parents the night before to let them know.) Lucy, who ran a licensed family child care home for kids from infancy through school-age, had brought some games (e.g., Connect 4) and cards (e.g., Old Maid). She told me she did not have Ariana in mind when she brought these items; she was just thinking that 90 minutes could be a long time, and some girls might need to calm down and do quieter activities. As it turned out, these additional options proved very beneficial to Ariana, who chose not to play on any of the McDonald's equipment. She involved herself for the entire time with the activities Lucy had brought. She was sitting on the floor, not in her wheelchair. At any time—without any prompting from the leaders—about half of the girls stayed in the area where Celeste and Lucy had laid out the quiet games and activities, playing with Ariana or with one another.

As for any other adaptations, either planned or spontaneous, they had been infrequent. At times, Lucy said, "we'll all do an activity sitting on the floor because she prefers that." It also went in the other direction. I saw them begin to seat the girls in a circle on the floor for a game, but then check with Ariana and learn that she would prefer to be sitting in her wheelchair. Without making a big deal of it, they told all the girls to get chairs and place them in a circle. Now Ariana's wheelchair did not separate her from the others.

At the Halloween party, they worried about how she would do an activity that involved holding one's hands behind the back and trying to bite a cookie that was dangling from a string. But it turned out she could do it from her wheelchair while others did it in a standing position.

Parental Roles

LaToya was always accompanied by a parent during her participation in the Brownie troop. The mother's or father's role, as I have described it, was that of a personal attendant, to provide hand-over-hand assistance on tasks such as arts and crafts or using a spoon to spread the tomato sauce for a mini-pizza, as well as to help interpret if LaToya was trying to express something with her Liberator. Martha also helped to devise ways of modifying the Try-It activities, which we shall discuss later in this chapter.

When Katrina first began bringing Erica to Brownies, she too remained with the group the entire time—sometimes sitting right with Erica, sometimes watching from another table. Just as she had told me six months earlier, she wanted to make sure she was comfortable with the leaders and confident the other girls would be accepting of her daughter. While she was there, she exhibited what appeared to be a thoughtful approach to how much to intervene. She seemed conscious of not overly interfering in the natural interactions with other girls while at the same time offering support.

During the color guard ceremony, which included the Girl Scout Promise and Pledge of Allegiance, Katrina helped her daughter stand in the right place but didn't worry about the fact that Erica held up the wrong hand. During a circle game, Katrina joined in and tried (without much success) to get Erica to run around the circle on her own when she was tagged. During a "secret code" activity that Erica could not comprehend, Katrina helped her draw some faces and a few letters of the alphabet with a pencil.

After the first few meetings, Katrina began leaving for part of the time, getting a few errands done (as she told me) and returning. In

January, the girls were invited to accompany their leaders to a theatrical production on a Friday evening at a high school in Brewster. For the first time, Katrina let Erica attend without her. It went fine. "The only thing that made it hard with Erica," Tammy said, "was when she had to go to the bathroom, and there's only certain times you can leave the auditorium during the play, with the crowd and everything."

Comparing the two mothers, Katrina played a different kind of role from Martha. She too acted as kind of a personal attendant at the very beginning but mostly provided emotional support. As time went on, she backed off. She was there in part for her own reasons, independent of Erica's needs, to assure herself that the troop was an accepting and supportive place for Erica. Martha had no similar need to establish the credibility and integrity of the troop leaders because of her prior association with both of them through the public schools.

Ariana's parents did not play any larger a role during meetings than the parents of typically developing peers. One or both of them wheeled her into the meeting space and immediately departed. One time, the downstairs room where their Brownie troop ordinarily met was taken, and they met upstairs instead. Her father carried her up, without her wheelchair, and the leaders had to carry her down and back up when she asked to go to the bathroom during the meeting. She was able to sit in a chair at a table, alongside the other girls, for the arts-and-crafts activities and the snack.

Jennifer's mother, Patsy, played an entirely different role from any of the others: She acted as sign language interpreter for her daughter. She had extensive previous experience as a Girl Scout volunteer, dating to when her oldest daughter was in Juniors, more than 10 years earlier. Because of this history and because the interpreter role would make it necessary to be present at meetings anyway, she became the assistant leader for Jennifer's Junior Girl Scout troop. Older sister Laurie also attended Jennifer's meetings about half the time, as her work schedule permitted. Sometimes she was there with their mom, and occasionally she and Jennifer arrived without Patsy. Whenever Laurie was present, she took responsibility for the sign language interpretation rather than her mom. Neither Laurie nor Patsy had studied sign language formally, but both had achieved some fluency. Of the two, Laurie was more proficient.

Volunteer Leaders' Perspectives

Francine told me that, even if she and Tammy were able to handle LaToya's mobility, communication, and other personal needs, they needed a parent there as a backup in case of a medical emergency. The following is from my interview notes:

The parent needs to be somewhere nearby. At the end of the second or third meeting, I was speaking with Martha, and LaToya was making a gurgling sound, and I asked her about it, and she said she seemed OK. Then it turned out she had a seizure that night and had to be rushed to the hospital. It's more for that reason that we'd want someone around. As far as the Liberator, we can be trained.

Regarding the participation of LaToya in the Brownies, the leaders communicated extensively with Martha. (This was easy to do, since both of them worked in the public school with one of Martha's other children with special needs.) Martha told me that at first, Francine or another co-leader would telephone her in advance to inform her of what activity they were planning to do and ask what kinds of preparations they could make to facilitate LaToya's participation. Generally, Martha told them not to bother, that she would be responsible for any extra materials or preparations.

The leaders had much less communication with Erica's family. In fact, Tammy and Martha had been very surprised when the parents dropped Erica off to go with them to the theater production in Brewster. They were pleased to be able to include Erica as a troop member, and neither of them told me they expected a higher level of communication from Katrina than they received. But I was left with the impression that they would have appreciated a somewhat greater level of communication and support.

Lucy and Celeste, co-leaders of the troop that included Ariana, did not feel that it had been difficult at all to have Ariana as a troop member. Not only did Ariana's parents not stay around (like LaToya's parents and to a lesser degree, Erica's mother). The leaders did not have even a telephone conversation with Ariana's parents prior to the start of the program year. They had a passing acquaintance with Ariana and her parents, because they each had daughters who attended Francine's troop with her the previous year and because Ariana's family and Celeste's family attended the same church.

One situation that reflected the lack of communication between the leaders and the family arose during the course of my observations of this troop. Lucy and Celeste realized they didn't know what type of support Ariana needed in going to the bathroom (e.g., getting from her wheelchair to the toilet seat and back). In the first few meetings,

Ariana had not asked about going, but they wanted to be prepared to handle it properly when she did. They conferred with each other and decided to ask the parents. The parents explained that she would need an adult to lift her up and back to her wheel-chair and nothing more. By their own recollection, that was the only issue on which they needed to seek information related to Ariana's disability during their first year as leaders.

Leaders Whose Own Children Had Special Needs

Lucy and Celeste viewed Ariana's inability to walk as a minor issue compared with other possible special needs. "It might be good to have a girl like LaToya or Erica," Lucy said. (Their own daughters had both been in the troop with LaToya before it was divided into two.) "Girls don't see Ariana's disability as any different from them. But having a girl with some other special needs would really help them in understanding handicaps." Celeste nodded her assent. Both stated that they would have been comfortable if the other girls with special needs had been assigned to their troop instead of Francine's. They thought they would have figured their way as they went along, just as they did with Ariana's more limited (in their view) type of disability.

Lucy and Celeste each had a child with special needs, and each in her own quiet way expressed strong commitments to the value of including all children. Lucy's daughter Nellie, who was one of the Brownies in the troop, took Ritalin. Although the medication was prescribed in connection with her ADHD diagnosis, Lucy made a point of avoiding the use of any label when discussing it with her. "She just knows that this medicine helps her concentrate."

Celeste was the mother of Cliff, whose work for the WPRD (tending to the tee-ball equipment) was noted in an earlier chapter. She had gone through the trauma of watching him lose substantial hearing in both ears after a high fever at age two and lose all the oral language he had acquired up to that point. Since age three, he had worn hearing aids in both ears. She was impressed (and even a bit surprised) at how well he had been coming to terms with his own condition now that he was a preadolescent. For instance, he volunteered to give a science report in school on the human ear and, in connection with that, to discuss his own impairment. There was no doubt that the experience of both of these leaders with their own children had helped to shape their sympathies to other children and families.

Celeste's daughter, Misty, was also one of two or three troop members that Ariana felt most comfortable calling on for assistance. And

Misty liked to be called on. ("Get me some glitter," Ariana would call out. "Please get me a scissors." "Could you push me to the other side of the room?) Celeste attributed this responsiveness to Misty's "little mother" attitude. I thought that growing up with her only sibling having a serious hearing impairment must have played a role as well in causing her to notice and be empathetic to other children with various kinds of special needs.

Gretchen considered Jennifer her "dream baby" and seemed to be very fond of her. When she had been pregnant with her daughter Sherry, she and Patsy were working at the same factory. She dreamed that Patsy was also pregnant—before Patsy had discovered the truth for herself. When both daughters were five years old, Gretchen started a Daisy troop, and Jennifer joined it. Sherry and Jennifer became friendly through Girl Scouting and had slept over at one another's homes. (As indicated earlier in this chapter, however, Jennifer did not identify Sherry among her best friends. She reserved that label for two of her Brewster school companions who were deaf.)

Gretchen did acknowledge some frustration in leading the troop with Jennifer as a member, but it was not with Jennifer herself. She did not think that discussions taking place during meetings were always as fully communicated to Jennifer as they might be. I could see that neither Patsy nor Laurie interpreted everything that was being said during meetings and that Patsy left out more than Laurie. Each of them tended to skip some of the comments of other girls during discussions while making sure to interpret the instructions that Gretchen made as leader. Gretchen considered the sign language interpretation to be Patsy's responsibility and not her place to comment on or criticize. (She had bought a book to teach herself signs a few years earlier, but had never gotten very far with it.)

I asked about the logistics of the seating. The troop sat around a long cafeteria-style table, with Gretchen at one end. Jennifer generally took a seat about halfway down the table from Gretchen, and then Patsy or Laurie seated herself either directly across from Jennifer or right beside her. When Jennifer was watching the signs from her mom or sister, she could not be simultaneously looking at Gretchen's speech or body language. Wouldn't it make more sense, I asked, to have the person doing the interpreting sit next to you, so Jennifer could see you and the sign language at the same time? Gretchen replied that this had crossed her mind, but because Patsy was not only Jennifer's mom but also the assistant troop leader, she didn't feel it was her place to comment.

COMMITMENT TO INCLUSION AMONG TROOPS IN WABASH AREA

Why did the parents of Erica, LaToya, Ariana, Jennifer, and Lindy find the Girl Scout troops in Wabash to be a generally receptive place for their daughters? There was no single answer to that question. The national organization had taken a stand in favor of inclusion, as well as other forms of what they called "pluralism." For a variety of reasons, many of the leaders who became active in Girl Scouts in Wabash were unusually sensitive to girls with disabilities and empathetic toward the particular girls who came along. Francine and Tammy worked in special education classrooms. Lucy and Celeste had kids of their own with special needs. Gretchen had worked with Jennifer for many years. Jennifer's mom and sister were active volunteers themselves.

Perhaps these leaders would have become active in the Girl Scouts and been available to work with these girls without any extraordinary efforts on the part of the local Girl Scout leadership. But in the years leading up to this study, two volunteer leaders had played an exceptionally strong role in moving the local Girl Scouts, in their philosophy and their practice, in a more inclusive direction. One was my initial informant, Rosemary, who had facilitated my contact with five families (including the parents of LaToya, Ariana, and Jennifer). The second was Mindy, who had become a staff member of the Girl Scout council about four years before the study was launched.

Rosemary's Encounter with the Boy Scouts

"It was one of my dreams that he should be a Boy Scout, like his Uncle Pete that we named him for," Rosemary told me, speaking of her son. When they were living in another state, Peter was saved from an episode of sudden infant death syndrome (SIDS) at the age of four and a half months because his father noticed him looking blue in his crib and gave him cardiopulmonary resuscitation. A helicopter ferried him to a hospital, where doctors kept him alive with the help of a ventilator. But even when he was able to breathe on his own and finally went home after 66 days in the hospital, the doctors told Rosemary and her husband that he would not live to see his new sibling. (Rosemary was pregnant at the time with her daughter Patty.)

The doctors' predictions were off the mark: Pete lived to age twelve and a half. He had visual and hearing impairment, needed a wheelchair for mobility, needed support to hold his head up, and communicated only by his eye movements, a few vocalized sounds, and some moving of his arms. But these limitations did not keep him from becoming a fan of (among other interests) televised sports. In the years before his death, according to his mother, he was an enthusiastic adherent of any sports programs that featured brightly colored uniforms and fast action; especially the state university basketball team, Sunday morning auto racing, and the Winter Olympics downhill skiers.

The family moved back to Wabash (having lived there briefly before) when Patty was six months old and Peter was 17 months old. They had remained in the area ever since. Like other Wabash children with severe developmental disabilities prior to the fall of 1994, Pete was bussed to Brewster for his schooling from age three until the time of his death. Although they lived in Wabash, opportunities for Pete to interact with other children his own age in his own community were almost nonexistent. When he was five years old (in 1987), a woman who was one of the volunteer leaders of the Cub Scouts in Wabash approached Rosemary and said, "If you eventually want Peter to be a Boy Scout, you should put him in Tiger Cubs now."

Because she had always dreamed of Peter becoming a Boy Scout, she took up the rare invitation with great delight and began to prepare herself and her son for the initial family picnic. From a nephew, she obtained a Cub Scout bandanna to put around his neck and dressed him for the occasion in a newly purchased T-shirt that was sold by the local Cub Scout pack. During the picnic, she pulled out his feeding syringe from her backpack and fed him through his G-tube. "The kids were OK with this, but the parents weren't."

She heard the feedback the very next day from the leader who had invited her. Several parents had threatened to pull their boys out if she let Peter join the troop. The leader went in turn to her unit leader to ask what to do. The unit leader advised the Wabash coordinator not to allow Peter to join the Tiger Cubs.

Greatly distressed, Rosemary's next step was to discuss the matter with a paid staff member at the regional Boy Scout Council. (There were approximately 330 such councils at the time of the study; the offices for the council serving Wabash and surrounding areas was in Brewster.) Their response was to offer to support Rosemary if she wished to start a special pack for boys with special needs. "But that's not the point," she told them.

She phoned her sister in California, who had a son completing his Eagle Scout requirements and who was heavily involved herself as a volunteer. "Can they discriminate like this?" Rosemary wanted to know.

Her sister advised her that, unfortunately, she thought they could, so long as they were offering the option of starting up a special pack.[2] Not wanting to dissipate her emotional energy on this, she did not engage the Boy Scout organization any further on the issue of her son's exclusion.[3] But nearly a decade later, the experience still rankled. "In Tiger Cubs, all the parents stay, anyway. I never wanted to just leave him there. I would have been with him!"

A month or so following her disappointing experience, Rosemary was approached by someone from the school that Peter attended in Brewster. They told her Peter was welcome to join their Tiger Cub pack. She appreciated the offer very much, but she had recently begun to work in Brewster, so "it would have meant me staying around town for an extra hour (while the troop met at Pete's school) and then driving home to Wabash afterward, which I didn't want to do after a hard day's work." (Like Martha 10 years later, she would have had to load and secure Peter and his wheelchair into a van and then unload him at the other end, in each direction.) It was the end of her contact (and Peter's too) with the Boy Scouts but a prelude to her later role with the Girl Scouts.

Two years later, Rosemary became active in the Girl Scouts. It was the second year of her daughter Patty's participation. First, she was a co-leader, then she volunteered to start up a new troop. "Once I was starting a new troop, I knew that I wanted anything I was associated with to not discriminate," she told me.

Fortuitously, Rosemary soon met Mindy, another volunteer who had also carried a similar commitment into her involvement with Girl Scouts. Mindy traced her sensitivity to children with disabilities back to her own days as a Girl Scout. In connection with a patch she wanted to earn, she took training with the Arc (at that time known as ARC, the Association for Retarded Citizens) that enabled her to baby-sit for families that had children with special needs. Subsequently, she studied therapeutic recreation in college and also became certified as an assistant for occupational therapy. Her own son had learning disabilities.

Focus on Ability Workshops

As an active volunteer, Mindy initiated a committee within the regional council that she called the Focus on Ability Task Force. Their underlying aim was to overcome barriers to the participation of girls with disabilities in Girl Scouting. Girl Scouts of the USA (Carroll, 1990), also issued a publication with the title, *Focus on Ability: Serving*

Girls with Special Needs, but the Executive Director of the regional Council told me proudly that Mindy "beat the national organization to it. She had her materials ready to roll out to our membership. And then, subsequently, (and, coincidentally, using the same name) they put out materials on the national level." When the national organization hosted a conference to kick off their new materials, Mindy attended it on behalf of the council. Three years later, she joined the council as a staff member. When I met her, Mindy was a membership specialist, one of eight full-time, salaried professionals on the staff of the regional council. The Girl Scout Council that provided services to Wabash was one of more than 300 regional councils chartered by the Girl Scouts of the USA. It was responsible for sponsoring Girl Scout activities in six counties. At the time of the study, they had 5,000 members, which amounted to approximately 17 percent of all the girls in the region who fell within the age parameters they served.

Rosemary and Mindy became valuable allies to one another. Together, they took the lead in planning and implementing the Focus on Ability activities. They had been doing this for seven years when I met them during the case study. They told me that the members of the Focus on Ability task force had started out with the goal of educating the entire community about people with disabilities. Secondly, it was geared to supporting and helping the leaders who had girls with disabilities in their troops. But by the time I met them, the energy of the task force was invested almost entirely in participatory presentations, called Focus on Ability workshops, which were designed to expose troop members to information about disabilities. Girls who attended the workshops earned a patch, which the task force had designed.

Each workshop featured one or more guest speakers with disabilities, who shared their personal experiences and knowledge, and interacted with the troop members. (As indicated earlier in this chapter, Martha got the idea to have LaToya join the Girl Scouts because the two of them had first participated as guest speakers at Focus on Ability workshops.) Brownies and Junior Girl Scouts were the age groups invited to attend the Focus on Ability workshops.[4]

Mindy had also become a trained volunteer for a puppet performance called Kids on the Block, featuring puppets who had various kinds of special needs. Two trained puppeteers conducted a dialogue with one another, using scripts that creatively introduced information about specific disabilities (one puppet was blind, another had cerebral palsy, and so forth), tried to remove the aura of fear and mystery from the subject of disabilities, and prompted the children watching to ask questions. Kids on the Block performances were incorporated into the Focus on Ability workshops.

From attending Task Force meetings, I saw for myself the enormous amount of organization and planning that was required for a few volunteers (no more than five or six, ordinarily) to organize these events. Among other tasks, they had to select the speakers, arrange for use of a public facility, disseminate the registration information to the troops, handle the responses to the registration, procure the requisite number of patches, prepare an agenda, obtain and transport the refreshments, and conduct the workshops. As a practical matter, they could not spend time on additional tasks so long as they were trying to organize at least two to three of these events per year.

Curriculum Infusion without Social Inclusion

I came to view the activities of the task force as an example of what Ferguson, Meyer, Jeanchild, Juniper, and Zingo (1992) called "curriculum infusion." This was one of three aspects of inclusive practice these authors encountered and labeled while conducting qualitative research in a school setting. Curriculum infusion meant making information about disabilities part of what children learned, (i.e., part of the curriculum). However, in the authors' study, the infusion of curriculum about disabilities came about naturally as a consequence of students who had disabilities participating as class members. And it came about simultaneously with the other two forms of inclusive practice, which they called "social inclusion" and "learning inclusion." Social inclusion meant developing a process by which other children could have social interaction with a peer with a disability (e.g., overcoming communication barriers). Learning inclusion meant developing ways of teaching the student or having the student participate fully in the specific subject matter or activity at hand.

The majority of girls who attended the Focus on Ability workshops did not have girls with special needs in their troops. Thus, they were getting a dose of curriculum infusion without the parallel exposure to the other two forms of inclusive practice. From what I could see, many of these girls did not make a direct connection between the information they were receiving and the possibility of having a peer relationship with a troop member with disabilities. After attending several Focus on Ability events, I concluded that curriculum infusion in the absence of the other two forms of inclusive practice made a very weak contribution to the future success of inclusion within the Girl Scouts. Without peers to further shape their views of disabilities, I concluded that the Focus on Ability workshop functioned, for many of the girls, more as a "focus on disability."

How Could Regional or National Resources Enhance Local Practice?

The Girl Scouts were way ahead of other organizations, locally, in the practice of inclusion. It came as a wonderful gift to families like those of LaToya and Erica to know that their daughters could be wholeheartedly accepted. There was no other youth program in Wabash that was inviting and encouraging the participation of children who had the levels of disability of LaToya, Erica, Ariana, or Jennifer. There was also no other organization in Wabash that had set up any kind of committee or task force to begin to address in a proactive way the inclusion of youngsters with disabilities, as had the Focus on Ability Task Force. The Girl Scouts definitely had placed the goal of inclusion on their agenda in a stronger way than any other local youth program. As Rosemary had vowed to herself when she became a volunteer leader, there was not going to be any discrimination of the kind she and her son had once encountered so long as she had anything to say about it. The commitment to the goal of inclusion was strong.

As for introducing any kinds of operational procedures to support the process of inclusion, it seemed to me they were still taking baby steps. In spite of the existence of the Focus on Ability committee, individual troop leaders—Gretchen, Celeste, Lucy, Francine, Tammy—were inventing their own inclusive practices as they went along, without benefit of the expertise or experience that others may have acquired, either locally, regionally, or nationally. They were figuring out, week by week, event by event, what kinds of support the individual girls needed. To the extent they turned anywhere for guidance or information, it was to the parents, and not to the Girl Scout organization. In fact, they didn't turn much to the parents either, except where there was a previous relationship between leader and parent on which to build (such as that of Francine and Martha through the public schools). Consider how little communication took place between Martha or Tammy with Erica's family or between Celeste and Lucy with Ariana's family. Consider that even though Jennifer's mom, Patsy, was the assistant troop leader for the Juniors, neither she nor Gretchen initiated any discussion with one another concerning Jennifer's experiences or whether they could do anything differently to ensure that she was successfully included.

During the time I was observing the Brownie and Junior troops in Wabash, I attended a meeting of volunteer leaders from Wabash and several other towns (all of whom were part of a single service unit), convened at a church in Wabash. In attendance were approximately 16 troop leaders, plus four or five other volunteer leaders who were part of what was called the Service Team. The leaders were mostly women in their thirties, with a few younger and older than that. I acknowledged that I had met several of them before and knew that some of them had accumulated important experiences in working with girls with various kinds of individual needs. I asked if any of them had had an opportunity to discuss these experiences with other leaders or staff of the organization. They shook their heads uniformly to the contrary. "Do you think it would be useful to share these experiences with one another?" I asked. They nodded in the affirmative.

I held up a copy of the manual, *Focus on Ability* and asked how many were aware of this resource from the national office of the Girl Scouts. Only Rosemary and one or two others from the Service Team raised their hands. Rosemary commented that members of the Focus on Ability task force each had copies of it.

One volunteer asked if the Focus on Ability task force would consider designing a new workshop—not for troop members but for leaders. She thought they could use some help in learning how to adapt activities and work on other aspects of inclusion. The fact that such a question was elicited among a group of volunteers—even granting that my presence was the stimulus for the question—boded well for the continued progress of the Girl Scouts in moving from the articulated goal of inclusion to the practical steps needed to undertake the process of inclusion.

7

"Sensei, Permission to Join Class?"

After I had visited the Karate School in downtown Wabash several times, I came to think of it as entering a world very different from the one that other local recreational and youth development programs inhabited. In this world, unlike the Boy Scouts or Girl Scouts, the uniform was not optional but mandatory. Instructors and participants were barefoot and wore a black or white tunic and loose-fitting, matching colored pants, the combination called a *gi*. Even though the instructors and the participants I saw were all American-born, Caucasian, and English speaking, they did not speak to one another in the language of free-flowing, everyday conversation. Instead, there was a stylized form of expression and much counting (and some calling of positions) in Japanese.

In this world, neither age nor gender nor status as parent or child gave a firm clue to a person's role. The oldest person there could be a student. One of the youngest might lead the group exercises. A child might be a spectator, waiting for and watching a parent in the class, or a parent might be the spectator, watching and waiting for her child who was participating in the class.

Leaders here helped participants to focus on goals that were more individualized than in the other recreational realms I observed. Leaders and students also had more physical contact with one another. In this arena, the social goals of having fun and making friends were not as central as in the others I observed. They were subordinated to intellectual and physical goals, achieved through practicing specific steps and body movements required at one's individual level of mastery.

MARTIAL ARTS AS AN ALTERNATIVE FOR YOUTH WITH DISABILITIES

It was Martha (whose daughter, LaToya, we discussed in the previous chapter) who first made me aware of the small, privately operated karate studio located in the downtown area. She said that her son Henry, who was turning 12 that year and had a mild form of cerebral palsy, was not able to enjoy playing on sports teams as much as he would have liked because of the way his disability constricted him. Henry was a boy with short, dark hair and slender build, a little smaller than average for sixth grade, who told me his favorite musical group was one that performed Christian rap.

His disability was not at all obvious to the casual observer—and surely not to his peers either. Martha described him as "an above average student." He did not use any type of adaptive equipment to support his mobility, was not involved in therapy, and had stopped receiving special education services when he entered first grade.[1] The invisibility of his special needs may have made it harder for him than for a more obviously impaired youth to come to terms with his limitations. "He's never been able to do other sports. He can't swim . . . he can't get it together to get things working the right way. He tried basketball. Riding a bike was a horrible time. . . . For the longest time, just when he'd be about to get it, it would be ice and snow and the bike would go away for another season. (He did eventually master it, at age nine.) He tried baseball."

Martha's experience watching him try to compete with peers in the athletic arena was so daunting that at times she said she had been tempted to stand up and say to other kids, "He has cerebral palsy—leave him alone!" Even the physical education class at school, she said, was a real challenge. Still, she and her husband had supported him, patiently, as he tried to compete in the arena of traditional competitive sports. "In basketball . . . he did not make the A team. There's also a B team; he was on that one, but he only played once or twice. He came home really upset."

In contrast, since he had started karate at age 11, Henry had achieved much more success, and his parents were unequivocally enthusiastic about the quality of his experience in that arena. The way

Martha saw it, karate was "a self-paced type thing, where you couldn't fail anybody" (i.e. let down the other players on the team). When Martha learned of an eight-week karate class offered at the Youth Recreation Center, she suggested to Henry that it was worth a try, and he agreed to sign up for it. He told me he liked it right from the start. He was surprised, among other things, by the fact that you had to learn to count to 10 in Japanese. But he did not object to that; in fact, he thought that it was "pretty cool." When the class ended, he began taking lessons (from the same instructors) at their private studio. (They charged a modest monthly fee of about $25)

Martha said she was reassured by talking to the instructors. They said they would hold Henry to the same standards as everyone else, but "if he has to do something 100 times instead of 25 or 50, we'll let him." She was also pleased that one of the senseis (the Japanese name for an instructor or teacher) turned out to be a nurse.

Since Henry began, the family had seen him work very hard at his karate, and it had paid off. He qualified for a state tournament, held in Chicago, during his first year and won a gold medal in one event and fifth place in another among boys of his own age and level. The first time I asked him about the tournament in Chicago, his otherwise impassive face broke into a proud grin. "My first time going to the state and I got a gold!"

A Second Participant with Special Needs

When I planned a first visit to see one of Henry's classes and meet his instructors, I was not sure if it would merit further observations. Would the fact that one boy with disabilities of a mild nature liked and excelled at karate necessarily indicate that there were salient lessons here for other families, for other recreation leaders, or for the readers of this study? Still, some of the contrasts that I noted in the first paragraphs of this chapter drew my attention and intrigued me right away. What cemented my interest further was the discovery that another youngster with mild disabilities was also a karate devotee and patron of the same studio.

Nicole turned 10 and entered fourth grade shortly after I met her. She had long, straight, dark-brown hair and a friendly but serious demeanor. Her family had come to Wabash two years ago from one of the smaller towns in the area. She was in special education for her speech impairment and motor delays, each of which were noticeable but mild. She told me she spent about half of each school day in a special education resource room and the other half in a regular classroom ("the normal class" was her phrase).

To talk to her, even briefly, was to recognize that she was bright, thoughtful, and had an unusually expansive vocabulary for her age. Her speech impairment was evident, however, in her skipping the *r* sound in most words where it appeared and also in what her mom described as "speech hesitancy." The latter took the form of the doubling of a vowel sound in the middle of a word, extending the word by an extra syllable. She typically did this in one or two words per sentence: *token* became to-o-ken, *place* became pla-a-ce. Her motor difficulties, which her mom described as a mid-range motion problem, were not readily apparent in her walking but became a challenge in sports and physical activities.

Like Henry, Nicole had started karate at the YRC and then signed up for a membership at the studio. Her parents gave her a choice between ballet (which was also taught at the YRC) and karate, and she had no trouble choosing the latter. She told me it was because of one boy she knew at the time, who had since left the area, who was "into karate." Her mom added that "she was also into the Ninja Turtles." (The latter were American pop culture icons among the school-age and preadolescent set of the mid to late 1990s—tortoises with attitude.)

Karate was Nicole's only involvement in an organized, group activity outside of school. She had been a Brownie, briefly, two years earlier, but had not enjoyed it much. She had also been a member of an after-school church group that she had enjoyed until it was rescheduled to a night that wasn't convenient for her and her family.

THE FACILITY AND SPACE

The karate classes were held on weekday evenings (twice a week), at a time when other nearby downtown businesses were deserted. The studio was located in a converted storefront that had been stripped of furnishings, except for some folding chairs near the entrance. These provided seating for guests or family members to watch classes or demonstrations and for students to take a seat during breaks. There were picture windows onto the street, and the name and phone number of the studio were painted in thick black letters on the window. Dozens of trophies, earned by the current and past students, lined the windows below eye level. There were more trophies all around the room and even more poking out of cardboard boxes.

The floor of the studio was covered with wall-to-wall carpeting, in shades of blue and green, without any obvious pattern. The walls did not look like they had been redone since the Karate School replaced the previous tenants (who had been some kind of retail merchants): They were a combination of pink paint, wood paneling, and neutral wallpaper. The walls were busy with posters, framed certificates of achievement awarded to the senseis, lots of photographs, and some news clippings. In a glass case not far from the entryway were two ornamental swords in sheaths and what appeared to be other art objects of Asian origin. On the interior wall at the back, opposite the entrance, a United States flag was draped. On either side of it were two flags I did not recognize. A teenaged class member told me they were from Okinawa and China. When the senseis saw this misinformation in an earlier draft of the chapter, they corrected it: The flags were from Japan and Korea.

Also displayed on the wall were all the belts, from white to black, that martial artists strove to attain. One of the teenaged participants explained to me that in the old days, one didn't change belts on achieving a higher rank. But the longer one was active, the dirtier (and thus darker) became the belt. Thereby came the tradition of moving up through the ranks from white to yellow to orange to green to purple to brown to black. (There were also intermediate ranks, created by marking the belts, so that you could have, for instance, a yellow belt with or without a mark, signifying two different ranks.) Depending on when students began and how hard they worked (and their natural abilities), some of the children had more advanced belts than some of the adults. In tournaments, one competed only against opponents of the same belt, the same age range, and the same gender.

BACKGROUND AND PHILOSOPHY OF THE INSTRUCTORS

The studio space was rented by Ted and Lena, a married couple in their thirties, who had lived in the area since the mid-1980s. They had other jobs during the day (he as a forklift technician in a factory, she as a nurse), and the Karate School was their avocation. (They told me their goal was to break even, financially; sometimes they succeeded, sometimes, not.) Both had taken up karate while in the military (which was also where they met). Neither had been an outstanding athlete in other realms, but they found that they could enjoy and master the martial arts forms with great facility. Both held black belts, the highest status one could achieve. Sensei Lena explained to me that there was no formal certification of martial arts instructors. Both she and Ted were certified as coaches and judges by the Amateur Athletic Union (which also sponsored many of the tournaments in which their students competed). But to determine the validity of any individual instructor's black belt, or to assess his or her ability to train others, the best way, she said, was to watch how well their students did in competition with those trained in other schools.

They articulated two goals for their students: (1) to help youth who may not be natural athletes to become good enough to qualify for the national level of competition, "even if they don't win anything, just to make it there"; (2) to promote Christian values. They started class with a prayer and tried to promote such concepts as "honoring elders," "treating others as you want to be treated," and "being honest—even if it means being honest about the fact that you didn't practice this week." They cited these as illustrations of how they were inculcating biblical themes. After Ted explained this during our interview, Lena added that they try to "keep it general," so that if a student were of a different religious background, he or she could still feel welcome.

Although their religious roots and practices lay in Christian faith, the specific karate form they practiced and taught had other cultural origins. The founder of the form, with whom they had studied, had been stationed all over the world (in the military) and had blended ideas and forms from several Asian teachers. Ted and Lena called themselves *senseis*, and were addressed as such by the students. They called the studio a *dojo*; a handout they distributed to students defined a dojo as any place of learning. It continued: "The boundary for the dojo is at the door. Students will bow-in at the door to enter or leave the training area." Students did bow as they arrived and at various other points during the classes. A student arriving late, after class began, would stop just inside the doorway, wait for the sensei to notice him or her, and give a little bow, asking, "Sensei, permission to join class?" Sensei would grant permission. Ted told me that in his own training, the sensei would require push-ups or some other penance before a student could join a class after a late arrival.

The same handout explained that "rei (bowing) is done to show respect to one another . . . is performed by standing at attention and bending deeply at the waist." It added that this courtesy was to be extended only in the dojo or at a tournament (not, apparently, if they encountered one another at the Dairy Queen).

A young American, Mark Salzman, who taught English and studied martial arts in the People's Republic of China in the 1980s, captured the intense personal commitment that can exist between a student and his or her martial arts master in this evocative passage (Salzman 1987, 86).

One evening later in the year, when I felt discouraged with my progress in a form of Northern Shaolin boxing called "Changquan," or "Long Fist," I asked Pan if he thought I should discontinue the training. He frowned, the only time he ever seemed genuinely angry with me, and said quietly, "When I tell you I will do something, I do it, exactly as I said I would. . . . Your only responsibility to me is to practice and to learn. My responsibility to you is much greater! Every time you think your task is great, think how much greater mine is. Just keep this in mind: if you fail"—here he paused to make sure I understood—"I will lose face."

THE CONTENT AND FORMAT OF THE CLASSES

Ted and Lena divided their students one night a week into beginners and advanced (the other night, all students were welcome) but never divided them by gender or age. On nights I attended classes (sometimes one class, sometimes two), the attendance was between 8 and 12 students; the age range was roughly 7 through 47. The gender mix was about two-thirds male overall, but on a given night, depending on who showed up, it could be half and half. The classes were usually about one-third children ages 16 and under, about one-third young adults from 17 to 22, and about one-third adults over 22.

I observed complete gender neutrality in the way the senseis treated their charges, and this was true regardless of whether Sensei Lena was present. (Because Lena worked various shifts at a hospital, Ted sometimes ran the classes without her.) Similarly, there were no discernible differences in the way the senseis treated students of different ages. They were gentle but firm in their interaction with every student.

Classes began with at least 5 or 10 minutes of stretching and group exercises, sometimes led by a sensei, other times by a student. Henry led the exercises during one of my visits. The exercise leader would announce a movement or exercise and then count from 1 to 10 in Japanese, as everyone repeated the motion 10 times. Senseis corrected the positioning of students (by verbal comments or by physical touching) as they engaged in the various kicks and motions.

After the exercises, there were other kinds of group drills. For instance, the block drill required students to use open-and closed-hand movements to ward off sensei's attacks with a large black block (made of foam rubber) attached to the end of a stick about one-foot long. He wielded the block with varying degrees of speed and ferocity, in accordance with the level of skill of the student.

The majority of the class time was spent practicing *katas*, a kind of fight against an invisible or imaginary opponent. Each kata had a specific name and consisted of the execution of a series of 15 to 20 movements, kicks, and thrusts, requiring a total elapsed time (when done proficiently) of perhaps 35 to 45 seconds. During practice, the senseis ran through the first three or four moves and retraced them until most students could manage them accurately, then added on a few more and slowly moved through the entire kata. Sensei Ted moved around enthusiastically, his golden-blonde hair dangling over his forehead, his black-rimmed glasses propped above a thick, dark-brown mustache. He punctuated the practice katas with commands to the entire group ("Stance! stance! stance!") and comments to individuals ("You're not quite turning all the way. You're kind of goin' so far and stopping").

Weapons, Shouts, Sparring, and Board Breaking

Some katas involved striking at the air with poles and were considered weapons (*bo*) katas. There were other types of weapons besides the bo (including the ceremonial swords in the glass case), but in my visits, I saw no one training with these.

The proper execution of any kata included, at certain designated points in the routine, the letting out of a loud shout, referred to always by its Japanese name, which sounded, phonetically, like "ki-aii." Sensei Lena once commented while Nicole was demonstrating the steps of a kata that "our best ki-aii-er forgot to ki-aii!" There was apparently no one correct way to do the ki-aii. So long as it was loud and rather high-pitched, you could create your own style of shout.

Sparring, which took place approximately once a week, was another important feature of the training and one which seemed to elevate the excitement level of the participants. The senseis would pair off students close in belt level against one another (not necessarily of the same gender) and would also sometimes face off against students themselves. These matches were highly disciplined tests of concentration and skill. There was much more stealthy, silent movement than actual striking or thrusting. The objective seemed to be to wait for just the right moment to make the correct motion that the opponent was not expecting and strike with a hand or foot to land a blow on an undefended part of the opponent's body. Senseis announced points when blows were landed cleanly and pointed out that certain moves would be ruled illegal in a tournament. No one got humbled or hurt in these matches (except for sensei, one time). No winners or losers were declared. They were teaching moments, an opportunity to integrate one's recently acquired skills into a competitive arena.

A final aspect of the classes that was noteworthy was the breaking of boards (*tameshiwari*), which took place less than once a month, at times announced well in advance and accompanied by many visitors and much fanfare. The students were responsible for bringing their own boards of one-inch pine and for deciding how many to break, from what positions, and with what parts of their bodies (elbow, foot, open hand, closed fist). The more advanced students set up sequences of breaks, perhaps breaking one with a hand in front, the next with a kick to the rear, followed by a spin to the side to execute a break with still a different motion.

Although the students all seemed to invest a great deal of energy and emotion into the performance of board breaking, there did not seem to be any real loss of face associated with failure to execute their planned breaks successfully. I noted in my field notes that:

Only about 3 of the 10 actually succeeded in all their breaks the first time they tried. Some completed them all with second efforts on some maneuvers. One (about 18 years old) failed at all of his setups and was setting up again after class ended, trying to give himself another chance. A couple abandoned certain moves—a young woman about 17, for instance, couldn't get one of the breaks involving a certain kick. And others—Nicole, for one—had to change to a different technique to complete what she attempted. She switched to her elbow after failing with her fist two or three times.

I asked Nicole later if she was disappointed. She said no, she just wished she had started out knowing she should do it with her elbow. . . . In helping Nicole, sensei Ted said something I hadn't heard since the Bill Cosby record,[2] that you don't focus on the board, you have to focus past it, not "two feet past it" as on the record but "at least that far past it," showing about six to eight inches with his hands. He said that when she practiced—and they all did trial moves through the air several times before actually going for the break—she was focusing past it, but when she actually went for the board, she was just focusing right up to the board and no farther. (In Bill Cosby's opinion, the problem was, the board was saying, "Oh, no you don't!")

On one of my first visits, sensei Lena was absent, and sensei Ted had to teach the class strictly through oral instruction but without actually showing any of the moves. Why? Because during a tournament a few days earlier, another martial artist with a black belt had cracked one of his ribs in a match for grand champions. He complained, smilingly, that it didn't make it any easier to repair forklifts at work. But it was not something he regretted.

The other students, even the young ones, understood on some level that the sport (or art?) they were working at was not only a kind of expressionistic dance but also contained within it the explosive power implied by their sensei's injury. With hard work, they could expect to focus the energy of their bodies and minds in ways that had never before been available to them. This, too, was part of the appeal of the karate studio, for adult and child, with or without disabilities.

Enlarging the Range of Recreational Options

Henry did not view himself (at least not in my presence) as a person with any disability or physical impairment and seemed to be struggling (according to what his mother told me) with whether he could be successful in more traditional competitive sports (specifically, basketball). He dropped out of karate for several months, after I first observed him at the studio, to devote his energies once again to basketball. For a second year, he played on the B team.

He would not acknowledge to me that his basketball experience had any downside; he claimed to enjoy karate and basketball equally. "They're both fun." From his mom's vantage point, however, his basketball participation was still charged with emotional anxiety. She was not surprised at the way he presented it to me. "After all, he's an adolescent male." To her, the availability of the karate studio (and of these particular instructors) as a different kind of arena in which to develop and display his physical prowess made a very important contribution to his sense of well-being.

Henry did return to karate after a hiatus and was able to get his mastery level back up in time to win a gold medal at his second state tournament. He seemed particularly pleased that his brother, in his twenties, came to see him perform (along with his father).

Nicole was the second of four children, and she told me, unprompted, that one benefit of karate was getting away from being "cooped up" with her siblings all the time. When she left the living room where I was conducting the interview, her mom assented and added to Nicole's statement. "It's helped her to stand up to her sisters and brother, to assert herself, to not get lost in the crowd. She's the only one in the family to do karate."

Nicole also spoke of being able to "walk away, if anyone teases me. Before, I used to say, 'stop it, or I'll hit you!' "

Nicole did not have any other sport or organized activity that competed with her loyalty to karate. For the time being, it was enormously satisfying to her. "Mom and dad thought it would help me focus more," she said. To me, that sounded like it could be a direct quote from them, rather than something deeply felt by her. However, I was convinced I was hearing her own voice when she told me, "It takes a lot of concentration to break a board. You don't want to mind wander when you're doing that!"

Nicole's comments helped me to understand how participation in martial arts instruction was different in some critical ways from the participation of youth in other recreational domains. The practice of karate (or any martial art) was not just another way of making friends and being part of a group. Rather, it was offering to those children who found it valuable and helpful a certain very specific kind of physical and intellectual discipline.

Although I did not see any youth with more severe disabilities in the Karate School, Ted and Lena expressed a receptivity to youth or adults with any kinds of special needs, unless the person needed one-to-one attention beyond what they were able to provide. One parent had come by with a teenager with Down Syndrome, they told me. They had encouraged the parents to sign him up, but they had not seen him again. Lena stated that in general, there were many kids who "warmed the bench" in team sports who could do well in karate.

Maybe they didn't fit in athletically, they were slower at developing the skills, or maybe they can't pay attention for nine innings of baseball or more than halfway through a basketball game.

In basketball, maybe you have three weeks for everybody to get ready for the beginning of the competition and that may not be enough for somebody. This is a year-round sport. If it takes four months to learn to throw a good front kick, fine, there's not as much pressure to keep up.

In tournaments, Lena and Ted had seen martial artists who had various kind of disabilities, including at least one woman who used a wheelchair who "does some of the best punches and blocks we have ever seen."

For every technique, we have a criteria, based on belt rank, for how well it should be done. Due to physical limitations, some people can't do it. We still require the knowledge level about how to do it properly. But sensei reserves the right to waive any requirement.

If a person is in a wheelchair and can't make certain moves, but if they have the knowledge to direct another person how those moves are supposed to be made, then they can advance [to the next rank].

Their openness to persons with special needs in martial arts was not out of the ordinary. The *Detroit Sunday Journal* on February 23, 1997, featured a lengthy story, "From a wheelchair, he strikes a blow to disabilities," about a karate instructor who was a wheelchair user. The subject of the article was a 48-year-old man, Tim Schutte, who was born with spina bifida and was nonambulatory all his life. He began studying karate at age 19 and began teaching in 1988. "It took him four and a half years to earn his black belt, something that just one of every 300 students accomplishes. 'Basically, I do everything the other students do except kick,' Schutte explains. He stresses that none of the standards were eased for him when he went for his black belt. In fact, he laughs, 'I got knocked out. I got kicked in the chin" (Christopher Singer, 3, 7).

It was easy for me to imagine a child with a more substantial physical, emotional, medical, or mental impairment taking part in classes at the Karate School. It seemed to me that each of the aspects of the experience that I highlighted at the outset of this chapter—its ritual and ceremonial features, the age and gender mix, and the focus on individualized goals—would have made it a welcoming place for youth with many different kinds of abilities and disabilities.

Rituals, Age and Gender Mixing, Individualized Goals

It was evident that both Henry and Nicole (as well as most other participants) took satisfaction from the ritual and ceremonial aspects of the karate experience: wearing the gi, the ranking system symbolized by the different colored belts, learning to count in Japanese, bowing, and addressing the instructors in a formalistic manner. What's more, neither of them minded that punishments were sometimes doled out; for instance, for horseplay, inattention, or dropping a bo. These, too, seemed to be built into the structure of ceremony, hierarchy, and discipline.

Over the course of the study, I saw Boy Scouts and Girl Scouts conduct their flag ceremonies and 4-H club members recite their 4-H pledge. They carried out these rituals dutifully but without enthusiasm. At the Karate School, in contrast, the participants seemed to have gained an appreciation for the ceremonial aspects of the experience. In the other youth groups, the youth undertook the ceremonies in order to get to the fun part of the agenda. In the Karate School, the entire experience was suffused with aspects of ritual, and they seemed to respond positively to it.

The age and gender mixing dramatically reduced the kinds of competitiveness that made team sports hard for many children and that caused many (even if they didn't have disabilities) to drop out. Nicole's mother, like Martha, said she had tried to gently steer her daughter away from team sports. Henry, at age 12, told me he got to pair off sometimes with a man who was 20 years old, and he felt really good about that. When I asked if it was OK to have people about my age (gray and middle-aged) in the class, both Henry and Nicole expressed a high level of comfort. "Even though they're that age, they can still learn," was the way Henry put it. "I feel like I can help them get along," Nicole said. (I understood her comment to mean that she could help them to improve their skills and move along to the next rank.)

The reason there was no need to segregate activities by students' genders or ages was that students worked on individual goals, within their own belt levels. Ted and Lena felt that the rank system provided a framework for mutual respect across ages and genders. "No matter your age, you know things that the level below doesn't know. Each person has his or her own individual niche. It's almost like you're not compared to anyone else because of different ages, different genders, and different ranks." I also noticed that at times, individual students (adults or children) decided to drop out for a few minutes and watch the others practice a kata. The senseis encouraged this kind of choice making and role flexibility.

AN INCLUSIVE PROCESS—EVEN WITHOUT AN ARTICULATED GOAL

I concluded that although Ted and Lena had never defined the inclusion of youth (or adults) with disabilities as an explicit goal, they nevertheless had a good grasp of the process of inclusion. In part, this was attributable to the fact that they were working with only a small number of students. They told me they would have to do certain things differently if they were in Brewster, or in any community with a larger number of participants. Splitting the adults from the youth would have been one of their first changes, they said.

Some aspects of their success seemed grounded in the nature of the sport, as I have indicated: its incorporation of formalized rituals, its use of ability rather than age or gender as an organizing principle, its focus on individualized instruction and support for personal goals attained at one's own rate of progress. Each of these was helpful and appealing to a child who developed at a different rate or in a different way from peers of the same age.

Their own personalities and personal values were also a contributing factor. They were a couple who prided themselves on modeling gender equality. They viewed their work as a way of promoting ethical human behavior. They looked askance on some others in the martial arts community whose only goals were making sure their students won competitions.

Although the Karate School during the period of the study offered a successful inclusive experience to only two children whose physical disabilities were mild, I concluded that the philosophy and practices these senseis incorporated made it a good arena in which other youth with more challenging special needs could also have experienced success.

8

Answering My Own Questions: Conclusions from the Case Study

Graue and Walsh (1995, 139) make this comment on the value of research that captures a close-up view of children and families: "To try to think about children without considering their life situations is to strip children and their actions of meaning. . . . We must think of children differently than we have in the previously dominant research paradigm. Rather than sampling subjects to represent a population, we must be fiercely interested in individuals, particular individuals. The focus of inquiry must become intensely local. The lens of research must zoom in to a shot of the situated child."

In doing the research for this book, I was fiercely interested in particular individuals. To the limits of my descriptive powers, I have introduced readers into the specific settings that I visited and have let them zoom in to see the situated child, to hear the voices of participants, family members, leaders of programs for youth in the community of Wabash. Among the children with whom readers will have become familiar by now are Carlton, a seven-year-old with cerebral palsy who played on a tee-ball team; Artie, a 15-year-old with Down Syndrome whose parents sent him to the Boys and Girls Club in Brewster; Erica, age nine, who had motor, speech and language difficulties, and joined her first organized recreational program (a Brownie troop) after I interviewed her mom; LaToya, also nine, who used a wheelchair and an augmentative communication device and was already a member of the Brownie troop that Erica joined; Jennifer, a 12-year-old Junior Girl Scout who was deaf; and Henry and Nicole, ages 12 and 10, who both had mild physical disabilities (combined, in Nicole's case, with speech difficulties) and enjoyed the challenge of being students in a small, private karate studio.

ZOOMING IN, ZOOMING OUT

Readers have not only encountered these specific children but have viewed them in particular scenes or events: Carlton, brightening into a wide smile when he hears his teammates chant his name from behind the backstop; Artie's younger brother, Curt, aggressively nudging him forward in the on-deck line of a kickball game; LaToya, moved to laughter during a Valentine's Day party by Erica's uniquely brazen social interaction style; and Nicole, breaking a board, but wishing she had started with her elbow instead of her fist.

To be able to appreciate and to interpret in a meaningful way any one child's recreational or youth development experiences has required acquainting ourselves with a cast of other characters. One of my tasks was to grasp how the thinking and decisions of various others impacted on or interacted with the child's experience in the youth program or recreational setting. This allowed me to achieve a multifaceted clarity that was not readily available to those most closely involved within the setting.

In order to understand Carlton's tee-ball experience, I gathered insights from his foster parents, Sheila and Steve; probed the thinking of Rhonda and Tracy, who coached him; and had several conversations with Drew (Tracy's husband), program director for the WPRD, who made the decision to permit Carlton to play tee-ball in spite of his age and who made his team assignment. To give depth and background to the decisions Artie's family made, I interviewed the parents, observed Artie at the Boys and Girls Club, and met with their staff. I also spent time at the Youth Recreation Center, got to know its director, Greg, and found that for many children, including some with special needs a little less noticeable than Artie's, it was a successful venue for inclusive recreation. I made many visits to the Brownie and Junior Girl Scout troops in which Erica, LaToya, and Jennifer participated; spoke with their parents and leaders; and interviewed some typically developing peers. Similarly, I watched the karate classes in action, interviewed Henry and Nicole, discussed with their parents why they had encouraged them to get involved, and interviewed the two senseis.

The lens of this study has been primarily turned on these local actors. It would be a mistake, however, to believe that we can draw interpretations or conclusions about any of these experiences with reference only to the children themselves and those peers and adults immediately interacting with them. Later in the same passage quoted above from Graue and Walsh (1995, 140), they emphasize another precept: "Data records are constructed in and of the local context, but those records cannot be interpreted without reference to their larger milieu." The larger milieu goes beyond those players immediately interacting with these children and even beyond the case study community. My aim has been to zoom in to the individual child and his or her surroundings, and then zoom back out in order to see the picture from a much wider angle.

I have tried to understand the operation of the WPRD baseball leagues, and the challenges posed to them by the participation of children like Carlton, in the context of historical trends that have shaped recreation and park programs since early in this century. The local Girl Scouts are part of a national youth development organization, and I have tried to take stock of the ways that developments at the national level interacted with developments in Wabash. With respect to martial arts, I have looked beyond the particular practices and personalities of the two senseis I observed to appreciate that there may be components of the sport itself that lend themselves to accommodating individual differences.

As I have documented the increasing participation of youth with disabilities in specific recreational arenas in one community, I have also traced out the possible implications such participation may have for the multiple constituencies who are living through these changes—not only in this one community, but in every community where similar changes are occurring. Only a few of these implications have entered loudly into the arena of public discourse. (Should a professional golfer with a disability be required to walk the course, even in great pain, as Ben Hogan once did? Or should he be allowed the use of a motorized cart?) Others have quietly worked their way into the minds of children, parents, and the operators or leaders of youth programs. (Should volunteer leaders be responsible for individualizing program activities and routines for those with health, developmental, or behavioral problems? Or is that the family's responsibility? Should we place the child who has special needs with other kids the exact same age? Or can he or she benefit from being grouped with somewhat younger kids, or in sports argot, "playing down?" Should program operators seek information from parents about the individual needs of children with disabilities? Or does such an inquiry risk being regarded as invasive and discriminatory?)

In the balance of this chapter, I shall zoom out farther and take a look across all the programs I observed, leaders I interviewed, and families I met. This will give me an opportunity to comment on what I learned about issues I have raised since the beginning of the book and to generalize about answers to some of the questions I have asked.

COMMUNITY ATTITUDES TOWARD YOUTH WITH SPECIAL NEEDS

The negative reaction that greeted Rosemary's use of a feeding tube with her son at a Tiger Cubs' picnic in Wabash in 1987 seemed, just 10 years later, like an artifact of a different epoch. Francine and her husband had been active for a number of years in the Cub Scouts and Boy Scouts as well as the Girl Scouts. The first she ever heard of the incident Rosemary described was when I shared a draft of Chapter 6 with her. She was saddened to hear that such a thing had occurred in her community, all the more so because she knew Rosemary and had seen Peter around the community. She wanted to know if I thought things were better now. I told her that I did. It was hard for me to imagine an incident of the same sort taking place anymore.

It seemed to me that Rosemary's insight at the time had proved to be accurate. She had taken some comfort from the fact that the Boy Scout troops in Brewster, where Peter attended school, were perfectly willing to include him (if the logistics had been manageable). She believed that when kids with more severe disabilities were attending the neighborhood schools in Wabash, then a boy with Peter's developmental differences would be more accepted by the families there as well. At the time of the case study, children with severe disabilities were attending the schools in Wabash, and it appeared that community acceptance had widened.

In heartening contrast to the story of the Tiger Cub picnic was the case of Skipper Walls, a boy whose level of functioning, since the time of his playground accident at age seven, was similar to what Peter's had been. He communicated with only a few vocalizations, needed people to push him in a wheelchair, and took his nutrition through a tube. Yet when his older brother, Billy, was in Webelos (in between Cub Scouts and Boy Scouts) the year prior to the study, the volunteer leader went out of his way to try to get the family to put Skipper in the troop as well.

Heightened Awareness of Persons with Disabilities

The exposure of the community as a whole to the needs of persons with disabilities had been heightened considerably in the years since the Tiger Cub picnic. Like everywhere in the country, the consequences of the ADA and other legislation that preceded it were increasingly apparent in daily life. Notably, youth and adults with recognizable physical and mental disabilities were increasingly visible as consumers, employees, and community members. I have described Bill, the former high school athlete, tooling around town in his sport utility vehicle, wheelchair in tow, and Keith, a young man with developmental disabilities, who had been given his own key to unlock the YRC and do maintenance tasks.

A minister I interviewed told me his congregation had "cut out a couple of pews" in their sanctuary to make room for wheelchair users. The bank president told me his daughter was a classmate of Gordon, the only user of a wheelchair at the high school. As far as he could see, "they take him as he is." His presence in a wheelchair, unheard of before Bill, was not particularly notable anymore—except, as another informant told me, when he tried to use a kind of lift mechanism that had been designed to allow him to ascend the staircase. (Gordon didn't like the fact that other students had to clear off the stairs and wait for him to be propelled to the top, so he mostly opted for the elevator.)

"What's Wrong with Carlton?"

In the recreational and youth program settings that were at the heart of my inquiry, I found that eagerness mixed with a bit of uncertainty was the prevailing sentiment, rather than resentment or trepidation. Children with mild mental disabilities or hearing impairments who participated in WPRD baseball and softball leagues in the most recent seasons had been treated as equals by peers and coaches, as was Sean, the 16-year-old with epilepsy. At the Karate School, nobody paid any notice to Nicole's speech difficulties. Maybe it was the dysfluency of her speech hesitancy in normal conversation that motivated her to shout out the Ki-aii with such gusto and to enjoy the patterned and stylized exchanges that were required in the dojo: "Yes, sensei!"

Of the various program staff I came to know, it was the volunteer leaders of the Girl Scout troops who were the most comfortable contending with the most challenging special needs among their members. Almost as remarkable was that other parents, whose daughters were the typically developing peers in these troops, made no comments and asked no questions about the participation of the girls who had disabilities.

One of LaToya's troopmates had been fearful of handling LaToya's equipment: This was the sole instance I came across of peers acting squeamish toward a child with special needs in any of the settings I studied. But even this experience had its silver lining. Subsequent to the meeting when the Brownies had been exposed to all the adaptive paraphernalia, this girl talked nonstop to her mom about all the things she had seen and learned at LaToya's. Curiously, I also learned from her mom that the girl's brother was a special education student who was assigned to special classes due to his learning disabilities and ADHD.

No one on Carlton's tee-ball team thought the brace he wore on his leg was worthy of public comment. Kimberly, our least athletically inclined tee-ball player, but one with an impressive, multigenerational fan base, asked me one time, "What's wrong with Carlton?" I paused for a moment, before I realized why she was asking. He had gone over to the sidelines to sit with his mom while the rest of the players lined up in batting order. "He has a nosebleed," I explained. That was all she wanted to know.

Parents Sometimes Not Ready for Inclusion

The cases of Erica and Skipper remind us that progress toward greater inclusion in recreational settings was not a one-way affair, with parents as the advocates, struggling to overcome the barriers placed in their paths by community organizations and programs. Sometimes peers and program providers are more than ready to be accepting, while the parents are the ones holding their children back from greater involvement. In an earlier chapter, I recorded in some detail the thoughts that went through Katrina's mind as she contemplated whether to enroll Erica in the Brownies. In the aftermath of my interview with her, she was able to get to the point where she did make the decision to call and arrange for her daughter to join. Skipper's mother never did.

Having Skipper attend Webelos would have been fine with his brother Billy; it was mom who was reluctant. By her own recollection, she had protested to the leader, a man she seemed to like and respect, "How can he do the badges?" He had confidently reassured her, as she told me, that "we can let him do things in a different way. He can still earn some of the badges." But she was unmoved by this appeal. She also resisted Charlotte's appeals to bring Skipper to the Fun Days that she organized on behalf of a local social service agency. These took place just one building away from where they lived. She knew Charlotte fairly well and seemed to like her. I was not able to get her to articulate the reasons for her resistance. Taking her son out to activities that typically developing peers (and her other son) attended was simply not part of her plan, regardless of the level of community acceptance. Perhaps this mother found it harder than other parents of children with disabilities because he had not entered the world with special needs or acquired them as a baby. Living in a cramped, deteriorating subsidized apartment, sitting on battered chairs and wearing second-hand clothes, it was obvious she had very little in the way of material possessions. But one thing she did have was seven full years of watching Skipper grow normally, before the shocking playground accident that had changed all of their lives so dramatically.

Kids with Problem Behaviors Not Viewed with Same Empathy

There was one notable exception to my finding that program leaders in Wabash were prepared to work with children with special needs. Antisocial behavior or inattention to rules placed children in jeopardy of being branded as bad or irresponsible and dealt with punitively. If they were below the age of eight or nine, their behavior might be tolerated somewhat, but above that age, kids risked alienating the goodwill of leaders and being asked not to participate.

If the child was difficult for others to get along with, or difficult for leaders to work with, it didn't help if the leader knew the child had a labeled disability (such as ADHD). Instead of becoming more empathetic because they knew the youngster had a diagnosed disability, a label of ADHD served in the eyes of some leaders as a red flag to make sure to give the child no slack and demand appropriate behavior—or else.

Among the youth who were given time-outs and suspensions at the YRC, it was likely that some were diagnosed with ADHD. Some may also have been assigned to classes for students with behavior disorders or learning disabilities in school. Others who got in trouble there at times, like Ginny Riley, had not been given labels or special classes but had been retained in grade. None of these distinctions mattered to those who were supervising them at the YRC, coaching them in the WPRD sports leagues, or providing leadership in 4-H Clubs, scouting, or at the Karate School. Regardless of how schools, doctors, or psychologists labeled and classified these children, the youth program leaders and recreation professionals I came to know did not view or speak about these children with the same level of sympathy they brought to children with medical, physical, or cognitive needs. Nor did they extend to these children the same inclination to go the extra mile if need be. (Obviously, this posture did not generalize to all leaders I met; for instance, it did not apply to Lucy, the Girl Scout leader whose own daughter had ADHD.)

Were leaders who had little tolerance for the behavior of these children prejudiced against youth with disabilities? Were they opposed to inclusion? Not exactly: They were compassionate toward children with other kinds of disabilities. They found behavioral challenges more threatening to their sense of competence as leaders and as authority figures than other types of special needs. Moreover, even if they had started with the presumption that the child was in need of help, rather than punishment, many of the leaders would not have known what kinds of adjustments they could make to be successful.

How One Troop Leader Succeeded with a Boy with ADHD

David was 12, diagnosed with ADHD, and taking Ritalin. He was brought to my attention by one of his Boy Scout troop leaders in Wabash as a very difficult troop member, one whose presence exasperated both his leaders and his peers. The leader viewed him as a typical case of why it was so hard to have kids with ADD or ADHD involved in community activities. I interviewed David and his mom, together, in the trailer park where they lived and got permission from both his scout leaders and his family to attend his meetings. David soon dropped out of this troop but not out of the Boy Scouts. He rejoined a troop in a nearby town where he had been a member before the family moved. I was able to observe his participation and interview his leaders in both troops.

I should not wish to make too much of what I learned from a brief inquiry, a kind of side trip compared with the more sustained observations I have described in earlier chapters. But in this side trip, I encountered compelling evidence that the level of David's problem behaviors varied, depending on how the environment he entered was structured and how others in the environment reacted to him and interacted with him.

The first troop met in a big, lofty barn and comprised about 14 boys. David's physical appearance was bulky, pudgy, and awkward. Every meeting started, informally, with 15 to 20 minutes of hard-driving basketball. David had told me that he did not enjoy this at all, and I saw that he participated in it without enthusiasm and without much skill. There was no coaching or instruction during this activity; the leaders occupied themselves with greeting parents and preparing for the meeting. They viewed basketball as free-play time, something the boys did on their own.

The balance of the meeting was run in a straightlaced, no-nonsense manner. David frequently engaged in off-task behaviors. When everyone was supposed to be practicing tying different knots with ropes, he was wandering to another part of the barn, hanging upside down, and playing with the ropes in an unapproved manner. His personality came across as goofy and a bit contrary, and the leaders called his name only to give him negative feedback. The other boys ignored him. I never saw him in a physical altercation, but I could easily see how his personality, his physical awkwardness and size, as well as a chip-on-the-shoulder attitude he projected would lead him to shove or knock into someone (or worse), without much caring about the consequences.

When I saw David with his other troop, he was considerably more engaging and tolerable—although still definitely a handful. A bearded Vietnam veteran named J.R. led a much smaller troop (only six to eight boys) and clearly knew how to humor David. If David said something gross at the first troop, and a leader heard it, he was reprimanded. J.R.'s response, by contrast, was to retort with something equally gross—and then get David back on task. He saw beyond David's challenging behaviors. "He has a vivid imagination; he's in his own world sometimes," was one of J.R.'s comments. (His mom had told me that in spite of his ADHD, he could concentrate on Nintendo for hours.)

J.R. described a problem he had with David a few weeks earlier. David had been boasting and threatening other troop members with kicks and thrusts, based on some martial arts lessons he claimed to have taken. J.R. challenged him to a fight. David then tried to get out of it, according to J.R., saying that "we don't do that in the Boy Scouts." "He was right. Technically, we don't do martial arts in Boy Scouts. But I got permission from his mom," J.R. told me, breaking into a smile, "to fight him." The duel was never consummated. But—attention deficit or no attention deficit—J.R. had gotten the boy's attention. He had done it in a way that asserted his own authority and still maintained a good relationship with David. David clearly thought very highly of him and was much more eager to go to Boy Scout activities after he switched back to J.R.'s troop.

What insights can we draw from this brief side trip? David brought the same baggage (his personality, his ADHD) with him into both environments. However, his more serious problem behaviors were produced in interaction with one environment and not the other.

Not all of the key environmental elements were under the complete control of the leaders: The smaller number of boys and the more confined space of the second troop definitely made it easier for J.R. to keep David focused and positively engaged. But the Junior Girl Scout troop I regularly observed met in the same high-ceilinged barn where David's Wabash Boy Scout troop met. Whereas the Boy Scout leaders left all the open space inside the barn just as they found it on arrival, I had seen the Girl Scout leaders set up tables and chairs and move them into different positions, in accordance with their activity plans for the evening. Some increased attention to defining and shaping (perhaps even decorating) the space might have helped David to keep his focus better.

Other elements of the environment were under the control of the leaders. In starting off each meeting with basketball, where David felt incompetent, oversized, and a loser, the leaders of the Wabash troop were perpetuating his inability to succeed with his peer group. In taking his goofy comments and behaviors seriously, they put him further on the defensive and increased his sense of social isolation. Their reprimands only made the chip on his shoulder get larger and increased the likelihood of his acting out in an antisocial manner. J.R. knew that underneath all that beef and bluster was just a 12-year-old who wanted to have fun, and who wanted to be part of a peer group—even if he had never been very good at it. His decisions and responses led David in a very different direction.

PARENTS' ROLES, AND HOW THEY MADE DECISIONS FOR (AND WITH) THEIR CHILDREN

Recreational or youth programs in Wabash were becoming inclusive, not due to their own proactive efforts but to the extent that parents of children with disabilities decided, (together with their kids) that they wanted their children to join up. This was equally true of the municipally operated programs of the WPRD (including the Youth Recreation Center); the affiliates of national organizations, such as Boy Scouts, Girl Scouts, and 4-H; and of the small, private Karate School.

In an earlier chapter, I took note of the different roles and levels of involvement of the parents of girls with special needs in the Brownie and Junior Girl Scout troops of Wabash. At the YRC, I never saw any parents who stayed around, unless it was to speak with a staff member for a few minutes. A large number of the youth arrived independently of their parents, and many others got dropped off, with their parents remaining in their cars. Nicole's and Henry's mothers only attended the karate classes when there were special demonstrations, board breaking, or activities in connection with students getting promoted to higher belt levels.

Wilbur was nine and had a disorder involving his facial muscles that she referred to as tic syndrome; he also had ADHD. His mother was told by his baseball coach that he would appreciate if she were on the premises during games and practices, even though his disabilities were quite mild. The reason given by the coach for this was that if Wilbur got hurt, the coach would not know how to describe his condition to emergency personnel or understand the implications of the medication he was taking. The mom did not seem to mind, although at times it caused her to have to rush between two different diamonds. (Her other son was a teammate of Carlton's, and tee-ball was played in a different part of town from the rest of the baseball and softball program.)

Although Wilbur was not allowed to take the field at practices until his mom arrived, he usually got there before her, biking over on his own. She had a factory job; sometimes she didn't get off until 6:00 P.M, and some of his practices began at 5:30. She also told me he rode his bike to and from school.

"So, he can ride to the field on his bike," I asked, "and ride to school, but he can't be at practice without you?"

"Well, the schools have a nurse." She went on to say that she'd be getting him a bracelet with emergency information on it and hoped that then people would feel more confident about responding if a medical complication arose.

Segregated Options, Inclusive Options

Aside from Lindy's family, none of the other families I met brought their children to Brewster for Special Olympics. But seven-year-old Carlton and sixteen-year-old Gordon each participated in one-week summer camps that were exclusively for children with special needs. Gordon loved the camp he attended, but he also stated that no one had ever offered him the opportunity to attend a camp that would be accessible to him but not designed exclusively for those with disabilities. "If it was offered to me, I'm sure I'd try it." He was pleasantly surprised when I told him I had just visited a Boy Scout camp that had been made accessible for leaders or boys with physical disabilities.

Artie had played at one time in the Challenger Division of Little League in another state. (This is a coeducational league for youth from ages 6 through 18, who have either mental or physical disabilities.) Artie's dad would not have been averse to sending him to a day camp for children with special needs. There was one in Brewster, but it was too expensive for the family budget.

If Artie's parents had sent him to a segregated camp, it would have been because they were confident the staff there had training and knew how to respond to Artie's individual needs—not because of an outright preference for segregated as opposed to inclusive experiences. Gordon's parents and Carlton's foster parents also elected to use segregated camps because there were no other appropriate options for camping experiences for their children, where they knew that the children would have the supports they needed to address their medical and physical issues. In both cases, they were also able to secure financial aid to defray the costs.

Other families did not seem to have considered using segregated programs (or to wish they were more readily available), with one exception. Patsy and her husband spoke somewhat wistfully of the town, three hours away, where the state school for deaf students was located. "Down there, they have enough girls to make a whole troop, just for the girls that are deaf." The remark was made in the context of the larger issues involved in Jennifer's friendships and social life. The parents recognized the tricky path they were on as hearing parents raising two (out of four) children who were deaf. "They get invited to parties with other adults—that we aren't even invited to!" their dad had chuckled. How much should they promote Jennifer and Colin's social involvement with hearing peers, and how much should they help them find a place in the deaf community? Like hearing parents of children who were deaf across the United States, they were far from resolving this difficult question.

Mom's Commitment Exceeds Leader's Expectations

Tara, whose reasons for keeping her son Brett from playing baseball we explored in an earlier chapter, did encourage him to join Tiger Cubs and then Cub Scouts. During Tiger Cubs, all the participants were expected to have a parent present, and Tara liked it that way. But she continued to attend the meetings after he advanced to Cub Scouts, although other parents mostly did not do so. She did not feel comfortable leaving him on his own. As with Katrina when she first brought Erica to Brownies, it was not the Cub Scout leader who required that she be present; rather, it was her own discomfort at the thought of leaving him there.

I saw that Tara still lived with the memory of the doctor she had described to me who had told her that Brett would never walk. Now she and her husband, Ray, were faced with making an agonizing decision about additional surgery for Brett. She was very committed to her son and very protective. Of all the parents I interviewed, she was the only one who shielded me from meeting her child (and me from meeting him). We had agreed that I would meet him if I scheduled a second interview, but I never did.

From her description, I concluded that her attendance at Cub Scouts was reaffirming for her, probably more so than for Brett. She took pleasure in watching her son engage in activities with other boys in ways she once thought (and still worried) wouldn't be possible. And she had been pleased and a bit surprised at the strong values that the leader promoted. "I got to know the leader, I liked his method. He promoted the philosophy that we're all different. I don't think it was because Brett was there, it's just his way. His own child has some kind of learning disability, I'm pretty sure. He's on Ritalin. I never asked because to me it was private. I think maybe it's an attention kind of problem."

The parents of children with special needs in Wabash were clearly continuing to take a greater level of responsibility than other parents did to ensure that their children could participate in youth programs. Yet the fact that Ariana (and, eventually, Erica) attended Brownies without having a parent present seemed to be a sign that this would not always be the case. For more parents to step back and permit children to participate more on their own in programs would require more communication between the families and the leaders.

Communication Between Parents and Program Staff or Leaders

The way Artie's father approached his son's enrollment at the Boys and Girls Club was unique among the parents I met: He was the only one who began planning, long in advance, for his son's participation in an inclusive setting. He visited the facility in Brewster twice, beginning several months prior to Artie's arrival in town. Admittedly, he had a more pressing need than other parents to secure his arrangements. He needed a place where Artie (and the two younger siblings) could spend their full days while he and his wife worked.

The level of his interest and his forthrightness about his son's individual differences made a positive impression on the leadership of the club staff. The early notice of his son's enrollment allowed them to plan for a springtime training related to inclusion. Also, they were happy to have the decision about grouping Artie with the younger children, and separating him from his brother Curt, taken off their shoulders and made by the father. If he had not given them these instructions, they would have assumed it was better to have him near his brother—precisely the opposite of what his father desired.

The staff started out cautiously accepting with respect to Artie. But they were used to picking up and dropping off most of their participants by bus and having very little contact with the families. So at the beginning, they did not relish the presence of an involved parent, possibly one who was going to be critical of them if problems occurred. But by the end, it was clear that they respected the father's involvement, appreciated his help, and liked him.

Other parents I met, despite their intimate familiarity with their own children's individual needs, were shy about making requests or providing guidance to the paid or volunteer staff of programs their children attended. They seemed to worry that they would be viewed as meddling if they provided such guidance when it was not specifically requested. Paradoxically, some program leaders would have appreciated more information and guidance but were reluctant to ask parents for it. They did not wish to convey the idea that they were fearful or prejudicial on account of a disability. The end result was that communication was minimal, even when both parties would have preferred more of it.

We saw that Lucy and Celeste knew nothing about Ariana's disability. They weren't even sure for the first few weeks what kind of assistance she might need if she ever wanted to use the bathroom during a meeting. Francine and Tammy would have liked to know more about Erica. They did not have the same kind of history with her in the public schools that they each had with LaToya. Katrina also told me that she had a few ideas she would have liked to share with Francine and Tammy, but she was appreciative that they were so accepting of her daughter and did not want to appear critical. Both parties wanted more communication. Both parties and the child would have benefited from additional communication, but everyone involved was being courteous and respectful—to a fault. As a result, useful communication did not take place.

They Belonged, Therefore They Joined

Like other local families, the parents of children with disabilities in Wabash watched the weekly newspaper for announcements of youth activities: meetings of 4-H clubs, registration information for sports teams or clinics at the WPRD, special events at the YRC. They received information about scout troops at least annually, when it was routinely sent home through the schools.

These parents made decisions about recreational activities for their children as casually as they did for children who were more typically developing. From the available options that came to their attention, they made their choices based on the child's expressed interests and convenience, knowing what others in their circle of friends or family were doing. If parents had played sports or been active in scouting in their own younger days, this played a part in shaping the plans they made with their children.

Thoughts about whether specific recreational activities or youth programs might enhance a child's skill development or social life were not uppermost in parents' minds as they helped their children choose an activity. They were not oblivious to these matters, but they placed no greater emphasis on them than if they were planning activities for a child without disabilities.

Sheila believed that it was good for Carlton to get out and run around and throw the ball in tee-ball. Patsy hoped Jennifer would make some Wabash friends through the Girl Scout troop. Erica began to vocalize more sounds and words in the months after she joined the Brownies, and her parents believed that her experience with typically developing peers in the troop had been a contributing factor. (She also had a new therapist in school, making it hard to know the exact source of her progress.) Wilbur's mother was delighted that he got invited to go swimming in the backyard of one of the boys he met on his WPRD baseball team. But it became clear to me that parents viewed these outcomes as welcome by-products of participation, and not the underlying reasons for participation.

The responses I elicited on this subject during my interviews led me to change the questions I was asking. For approximately the first five interviews with parents in Wabash, one of the areas I actively tried to probe was the kinds of social or learning goals that parents had in mind when they enrolled their youngsters in recreational programs. I was anticipating some reference to increased use of language in natural settings with peers who had no special needs, opportunities to engage in gross-motor or fine-motor activities, improved social relationships, or perhaps sensory stimulation. It became clear that these were not paramount considerations for the parents, and my asking these questions created awkward moments in which they became a bit defensive. The impression that I expected them to have specific educational goals in mind did not endear me to them or contribute to the kind of trusting, relaxed atmosphere that I wished to cultivate. Therefore I stopped raising these issues in a direct way and listened instead for indirect clues about whether the social or educational outcomes were part of what motivated parents to enroll their kids in these programs.

I came to see that enrollment of their children in typical youth programs was a statement by parents that their children belonged and were part of the community, just as much as any other child. If their children were in special education, they did not view these community activities as extensions of the children's educational plans. Indeed, parents I met did not seem to view the programs as "inclusive" but simply as the ones that were there for all children. They considered it customary for kids of this age to join these kinds of activities. They signed up their children because they knew someone else who was signing up or because it sounded fun or because they thought the child needed some structure in her or his leisure time (a preference that might have applied equally to a child who was more typically developing). Outcomes, learning goals, measures of success, costs and benefits, assessments of progress? Those were not the way parents in Wabash thought about the decisions and choices they and their children made.

The exceptions (the parents who hesitated to sign their children up for any activities) proved the rule. Katrina, at the time I first met her, was not yet really convinced that her child was entitled to be viewed as a member of the community, like any other child her age. By the end of the study, she was closer to that perspective. Tara had similar worries about whether her Brett could be viewed as just another boy in Tiger Cubs and Cub Scouts. Skipper's mom, still reeling from the unhappy circumstances in which her son found himself, also seemed not to think of him as belonging, in spite of the encouragement she received from the Webelos leader and from Charlotte. (Uprooted from her hometown by Skipper's accident, I concluded that in this community, she did not feel a strong sense of belonging, either.)

Jody was a parent I turned to as a resource from outside the case study community. She was professionally involved in delivering services to families with disabilities in a nearby county and also had three daughters active in community sports and recreation, one of whom, Andrea, had Down Syndrome. "To this day," she told me, commenting on her daughter's former participation in sports teams and a local choir, "we'll walk through the mall, and people will be saying 'hi' to Andrea, and I don't have a clue. I mean, you know, I'm just her mom. You know, along for the ride. They all know *her*."

Like Jody, the parents I met in Wabash looked to youth, sports, and recreational settings as places where their children could experience membership in the community. To believe that "my kid is known in this community"—and that he or she was accepted as someone who belonged there—was an aspiration nearly all of them shared.

THE CHALLENGES THAT FACED PROGRAM LEADERS

Sarah had been co-leader with Francine, of the Brownie troop that included Ariana and LaToya, before the Brownies were subdivided into two troops. When I met her, she was the Girl Scout troop consultant for the entire Wabash area. I asked her about any prior contact with children with special needs. She replied that the oldest of her three daughters had been in a troop with Lindy and that she had also gotten to know Lindy through school.

What insights had she gained from seeing how Lindy participated in school and in scouting? "The main thing I got out of it was that they treated her like she was normal. That's the one thing that sticks in my mind. And that's always what I've tried to do. I do the same with the girls that are in our troop."

Sarah's statements accurately captured the level of development of inclusive practice in Wabash among most professionals and volunteers responsible for day-to-day program delivery—not only in the Girl Scouts but among all the programs and activities I observed. They had a strong commitment to the goal of inclusion. But most shied away from what I have called (following Schleien and his co-authors) the process of inclusion.

Modifying Equipment, Routines, or Activities

In their book, *Integrated Outdoor Education and Adventure Programs*, Schleien, McAvoy, Lais, and Rynders (1993, 111) describe five types of adaptations that allow people with disabilities to participate in outdoor recreation and sports. Their typology offers a useful way to look at the activities I observed in the case study community:

1. Material adaptations (e.g., to gather seeds, use a large plastic pail instead of a small dish)
2. Procedural and rule adaptations (e.g., to gather pond samples, work from a dock rather than the edge of a pond, and have everyone wear personal flotation devices such as lifejackets)
3. Skill sequence adaptations (e.g., before a snowshoe hike in the woods, put on the snowshoes indoors)
4. Environmental modifications (e.g., make walking paths hard-surfaced rather than graveled)
5. Lead-up activities (e.g., learn to paddle in a swimming pool before canoeing outdoors).

The concept (and the lexicon) of program or environmental modifications had limited currency among the youth, family members, and activity leaders in Wabash. Of all the venues I observed, the Brownie troops were the ones where I saw the most examples of conscious reflection by leaders and parents about the individual needs of youngsters with disabilities and how to take them into account in the planning and implementation of activities. (This was also the venue in which the children with the most challenging disabilities that I saw were participating.) Even in this arena, however, modifications were occasional rather than incorporated into week-to-week practice. I described some of the ways that Martha helped to design Try-It modifications for LaToya and how Lucy and Celeste subtly altered their meeting plans at times, with Ariana's use of a wheelchair in mind.

Martha, with more than one child in special education, and Francine, a special education teacher when she wasn't a Girl Scout or Boy Scout volunteer leader, were among the few respondents I met who were familiar with the concepts of program or activity adaptation. Leaders who lacked familiarity with these concepts, however, sometimes responded to individual needs in ways that were consistent with the ideas articulated in the professional literature. In an earlier chapter, I noted one example of a material adaptation: the batting helmet adapted to keep Cliff's hearing aids from whistling. I also discussed the rule on "playing down" that was often applied to youth with special needs, although it was conceived with the red-shirting issue in mind.

This could be regarded as a kind of administrative adaptation for children with differing abilities.

Tee-ball, in its total conception, can be viewed as a "lead-up" activity for baseball or softball. Coach-pitched baseball or softball is a lead-up for the player-pitched version of either game. I also learned that the Girl Scouts organized overnights in secure, familiar, indoor facilities, prior to taking their charges camping in the outdoors: another form of lead-up activity.

At the YRC, I did not see any examples of modifications consistent with any of the categories outlined in the Schleien et al. (1993) typology. However, Greg shared with me his idea of making the sign-in sheet accessible if a member who used a wheelchair decided to join. I would view that as example of an environmental modification.

At the Karate School, I saw no examples of specific adaptations, but the senseis talked about competitors in tournaments they had watched whose routines were significantly modified due to disabilities. They spoke without hesitation about how they could modify routines if more students with disabilities (or students with more challenging disabilities than Nicole's or Henry's) came to their studio for instruction. They explained how, in subtle ways, they implemented modifications in working with Henry and Nicole.

We cannot allow Nicole to spar in a tournament setting yet. It's a coordination thing, for the sake of safety. We let her spar in the dojo, it's a controlled environment. Other students will slow down so they don't injure her. But in a tournament, someone could make a nice, high side kick to her and she will have no chance to react. . . . When she front kicks, she doesn't get her toes out of the way. They should be flexed (she shows me) but if she comes up against something hard, with them pointed straight ahead, that's a problem.

I concluded that although modifications and adaptations to meet the needs of individuals with differing abilities were by no means prevalent in the day-to-day practice of youth program and recreation leaders in the case study community, neither were these ideas completely alien to the way that volunteers and professional staff went about their responsibilities. At one time or another, most of them had the experience of implementing (or at least, as in Greg's case, thinking about) an adaptation in materials, routine, or environment to meet an individual's needs.

In contrast to the settings that I observed was a camp that Gordon described to me. Among the features he told me about were a specially built dock with a guard rail so he could fish without wheeling off into the water, boats that were accessible to his wheelchair, and video games and marshmallow roasts with adaptive seating. It was apparent to me that the widespread knowledge of adaptations that made specialized camping and therapeutic recreation possible had not yet been transferred to the inclusive settings that I was observing.

Rule Changes in Team Sports

The bank president I interviewed had four children of elementary through high school age, and he told me he had coached in the WPRD leagues for each of the 11 years he had lived in Wabash. He did not have much personal contact with families whose children had special needs, and none that he knew of had played on his teams. Still, he insisted that he would have tried his best to work with any youngster who came his way. He had the impression that most other coaches would be equally happy to include a boy or girl with a disability. "And Drew knows the coaches," he added, "and knows who to assign them to." He could imagine that some parents of children with disabilities were holding back, not signing up their children but only because they didn't realize "how much understanding would be shown."

He was only partly right. The reason that Henry's and Brett's parents were holding them back was not for fear of insensitive coaches. Rather, they were anticipating the unhappy feelings their children might come away with if they tried to compete but did not have the same ability level as peers—even assuming the coaches (and other players, too) were supportive.

So long as learning and fun were emphasized above competition, as in tee-ball, there seemed to be no problem. But the goals of learning and fun receded as children aged and moved into higher leagues. The WPRD eliminated tryouts from its baseball and softball leagues, minimized the role of All Star teams, and tried to jawbone coaches into conducting their practices and games in the least stressful and most fun manner for the young athletes. Still, there was a strong ethic of competition that no one seemed to know how to constrain. Unless one's disability interfered only minimally or not at all with athletic performance (as was the case with 16-year-old Sean's epilepsy), it was hard for any child with special needs to remain involved in the competitive sports leagues beyond ages 9 or 10.

Parents of children with disabilities in Wabash were going to have to continue, year by year, to decide (with their children) what the best decision would be: to play down, to play with chronological peers even if they weren't on the same athletic level, or to find another, more suitable activity. Even with a great deal of goodwill within the WPRD, there was no really clear process that was leading toward expanded participation of children with special needs in the area of team sports.

BEYOND ACCEPTANCE—TO SOCIAL INTERACTION AND FRIENDSHIP?

Because many of the children with special needs were in separate classrooms for much or all of their school time (and Jennifer was bussed to a different school district), the youth programs and recreational settings offered some of their only opportunities to interact with more typically developing peers in a group. Yet the leaders and supervisors of programs and activities I observed never focused in a conscious way on supporting children's social interaction or helping them to make friends. The energy and time of coaches were taken up with drilling on skills, teaching the rules, rotating players through different positions, keeping track of batting orders, and making smooth transitions between innings. The staff at the YRC were on the alert for behavior problems, responding to members' requests for equipment, greeting arriving members or parents, answering the telephones, or joining in some hoop shooting. Leaders of 4-H clubs, Boy Scout and Girl Scout troops, Boy Scout camp, and Fun Days were preoccupied with dues collections, planning, and decision making for future activities, organizing and supervising crafts, games, cooking, and other small group activities. At the Karate School, the senseis were entirely engaged in their instructional tasks.

The ways in which the leaders directed their attention and used their time were appropriate, even indispensable. But in failing to see the fostering of peer relationships as a part of their mission, they missed opportunities at times, or even jeopardized naturally occurring opportunities that could have helped children achieve a greater sense of social inclusion and belonging. Unintentionally, they sometimes undercut the quality of the experience for certain children with special needs.

Fostering Social Interaction—or Jeopardizing It?

I observed Artie in the game room at the Boys and Girls Club for close to an hour with the age group to which he was assigned, the 11- to

12-year-olds. For the longest portion of that time, he was watching or playing Nintendo. "Awesome!" he would yell to himself, thrusting his fist into the air as he operated the controls enthusiastically. "Yes! Yes! I got 'im!" "Aaagh," he said, with his hands placed on his forehead in agony. Meanwhile, a staff member passed wordlessly through the area every 10 minutes or so. Several girls and boys interacted with Artie and encouraged him intermittently, but one boy sat with him for the most extended period of time—at least 15 minutes. Eventually, during one of his casual walks through the game room, the staff member noticed the boy. "What are you doing in *my* room?" he asked, rhetorically. The boy left immediately for the gym, where kids in his age group (9 and 10) were supposed to be. Fortunately for Artie, the boy was not the only one who was interested in him. But even if he had been, I was certain it would not have altered the leader's action. He would have placed compliance with the rules above the value of helping Artie to feel socially included.

Another day, I was having a conversation with a part-time staffer at the YRC, a young man of college age, while he and I watched a group of 20 youth shooting around on the basketball court. One of the few girls on the court at that time, who was also one of the younger players (about eight years old) kept coming over to ask him for help with one thing or another. "Could you get me another ball?" "She took my ball away." "He's not letting me get the rebound." The staff member responded to her each time in a friendly way but grew increasingly short in his responses. What he did not see was that her persistent demands were a series of excuses to get attention from him, where none was forthcoming from peers. She had not succeeded in engaging the attention or friendship of any of the other players.

Earlier in this book, I described how Grace (Francine's 16-year-old daughter) lacked foresight in dividing the girls into three groups by counting off, inadvertently leaving her sister Annie in a group that consisted only of herself, both girls with disabilities, and me. In the same episode, I described how I offered my seat to Erica so that she could be closer to LaToya and more easily interact with her, rather than sitting all the way around the other side of a long table while we were decorating hats. I had to be assertive to get Grace to accept this suggestion. Her own inclination was to return Erica to her original seat because her attention was on the task and on getting the kids to comply with her instructions, and not on the peer interaction.

In each of these examples from the Boys and Girls Club, the YRC, and a Brownie troop, we see staff members or volunteers doing their jobs responsibly, as they understood them. But the fostering of positive peer relationships or helping children make friends was not uppermost in their minds—if indeed, they had thought about it at all. Consequently, they missed valuable opportunities, and some children were not as fully or successfully included as they could have been.

When Francine read an earlier draft of this book, she expressed appreciation for getting to read my narrative of that episode. She told me she planned to speak with Grace about the need to be more thoughtful when she divided the group in the future, to pay attention to which girls were getting into which groups, and to be supportive of positive peer relationships, especially when they involved the girls with special needs.

Keeping Children with Their Own Age Groups—or Not

In the settings I visited, it appeared to me that several of the children with special needs benefited from social interaction opportunities with younger peers without disabilities. Sixteen-year-old Gordon described his best friend—one who golfed while Gordon drove the golf cart—as someone in a younger grade. Carlton fit in well with a tee-ball team, although he was one to two years older than his teammates. Erica and La-Toya seemed to prosper as Brownies, even though they too were two years older than most of their troop mates. In the neighborhood where I grew up, it was younger girls—not the ones Laurel's own exact age—who would knock on our door to play with my sister.

My experience in the case study community then—together with my personal biases from knowing Laurel's history—inclined me to conclude that youth with special needs could benefit from involving themselves with younger peers. But I also encountered evidence that youth with special needs benefited from having older youth, or even adults, as peers in recreational settings. Lindy had taken pride in her interactions with adult Special Olympians. Gordon spoke to me of the camp he attended, where he stayed in a cabin with boys and young men with disabilities, spanning ages from 12 to 20. There were adult campers who were considerably older than that who were also involved in activities with him. I was intrigued to hear how enthused Gordon was, how much he was looking forward to going back for his eleventh year to the same camp. The fact that other campers had disabilities much different from his seemed to be part of the fun. "You're accepted there if you wear glasses or if you use a walker or have a speaking device . . . or if you're 'hyper.'"

I felt perplexed as I tucked away my notes and my thoughts after completing the interview with Gordon. From my reading and discussions over the years with other advocates of inclusive philosophy and practice, I was inclined to question why children and adults would be placed together in a camp just because they all had disabilities. After all, typically developing 12- or 14-year-olds would never be assigned to a cabin with 20-year-olds, unless the 20-year-old was a counselor. Nor would their parents send them off to a camp where they would be mixing in with adults, unless it was a family camp in which the parents were also participating. However, it was obvious to me that Gordon found the camp to be a wonderful place, and the age mix seemed to be part of the attraction.

Soon after, I found myself in the Karate School. As described in an earlier chapter, I watched adults and children, from ages 7 to 47, participating together. I experienced it as a very liberating atmosphere, freeing children and adults from expectations based on factors other than individual ability. Ted and Lena acknowledged that mixing ages was not a conscious part of their philosophy; rather, it was an artifact of opening a martial arts studio in a relatively small community where there weren't enough paying customers to justify separate classes for children and adults.

I sensed that not only Henry and Nicole, with their special needs, but all the youth who participated, gained from the multigenerational nature of the experience. They were learning and exercising along with people who were old enough to be their parents or grandparents. Looking around, they could see belts of different colors, which bore no correspondence to the ages, sizes, or genders of the person wearing the uniform. They were each provided individualized feedback and each valued, as an individual, not as an age group.

This led me to review in my mind what Gordon had told me about his camp. Perhaps, in a place where disabilities were no longer a strongly distinguishing characteristic (because every camper had one or several), he was able to feel respected as an individual. Perhaps no one else had the same combination he had of age, gender, use of wheelchair, and high level of cognitive and language skills. Perhaps, like the students in the Karate School, he felt that at camp, his deficit (not walking) was overlooked, and he was measured only against himself.

In the fields of early intervention and special education, we use terms such as natural environments and normalized settings to refer to the practices that are commonly associated with more typically developing peers. Advocates of inclusion usually take the position that these natural or normalized arrangements are the ones that are most desirable for persons with disabilities as well. But what if the society has adopted certain practices that are ill-suited to meeting developmental needs? Did being "normal" make all the manifestations of the world of typically developing peers better? In the area of generational mixing, it seemed to me, there was room for the "typical" world to learn something from the experiences of Gordon and Lindy.

Siblings

At least half of the active members at the YRC arrived with siblings, and most of them played together if they were close in age (within two to three years) and of the same gender. It would be natural if the staff saw a new member with disabilities arrive with a sibling (particularly one close in age and of the same gender) to encourage them to find things to do together.

The staff of the Boys and Girls Club in Brewster told me that were it not for the parents' idea to separate Artie and his brother, they certainly would have put them together in one group and relied on Curt to help them communicate with Artie. But as we have seen, in that family, there were important reasons not to do that.

Staub, Schwartz, Gallucci, and Peck (1994) studied the friendships of four pairs of students with and without disabilities, all attending the same school, ranging from kindergarten to grade six. One theme that these relationships had in common was that "as the friendships developed, the students without disabilities took on some responsibility for their friend with disabilities. Except in [one] case, teachers began to count on the children without disabilities to help their friends with disabilities" (323). Later (324), the researchers ask "whether or not there is a tension between the role of being a friend and being a tutor or caretaker. What are the benefits and disadvantages of both of these roles? What do these roles look like, and are students able to move in and out of these roles at different times and in different activities during the day?"

The family dynamics we viewed in Artie's family raise similar questions as applied to siblings, rather than unrelated friends. From what I observed, Curt was able to move in and out of his caretaker role, but it seemed that his playing that role, even part of the time, may have interfered with his ability to make friends with other program participants. For instance, when he was focused on making sure that Artie moved up to the front of the lineup so he would get a turn to bat, he was oblivious to how he was coming across to the other boys involved in the game. His role as guardian and protector of his brother superseded in that moment any effort to nurture personal relationships.

We cannot conclude from this one instance that all siblings in comparable circumstances (one with special needs, one without) will benefit from being separated. Some families may want the more typically developing sibling to help in interpreting behavior or communication. Others may want them to be kept apart. Still others will not have given it much thought, and the responsibility for thinking through the pros and cons of how to group siblings will fall on the program leaders. What we learned in Wabash should be enough to alert recreation and youth program supervisors to the fact that past experiences with families of typically developing children will not always fully prepare staff and volunteers for the issues that arise when a young person with disabilities is part of the family. Extra thinking, planning, and communicating with the family in these situations—even if the parent does not take the lead in initiating it—may lead to greater success for the kids and the program leaders.

THE INFLUENCE OF MY RESEARCH ACTIVITIES

Katrina told me that she would not have signed up Erica for Girl Scouts during the year I was conducting the case study if I had not interviewed her. (She might have gotten around to it eventually.) It was the information I shared with her during the interview, about other girls with special needs who were currently participating in the local Girl Scouts and the fact that parents were always welcome to attend troop activities, that spurred her to follow through on it sooner rather than later.

After reading a draft of the section of this book covering her own Brownie troop's activities, Francine reflected on the social grouping and social interaction issues I raised. In my presence, she began discussing these matters with Tammy, her assistant both at school and in the troop. For her part, Tammy wrote me a note after reading the same draft material, thanking me for sharing it, and stating that as a result of having read my descriptions and interpretations, she had some new ideas. Part of her note said, "I should have taken LaToya to where the other girls were" during the snack time at the conclusion of the Valentine's Day party. I did not necessarily agree with her conclusion. What I did see, and thought was good, was that Tammy was more aware of the implications of whatever decisions she made on the social interactions among the girls in the Brownie troop.

The bank president I interviewed, who was also an officer for a child welfare foundation, acknowledged that at present, local business leaders in Wabash were well aware of the need to extend a hand to enrich the recreational options of youth from low-income backgrounds. But no one had ever before drawn his attention to the need for expanded recreational options for youth with other kinds of special needs. In answer to a suggestion I made, he said, "Sure, if Greg told us that there was a need to bring somebody on staff a few hours a week [at the YRC], to help figure out how to address unmet needs of kids with disabilities, it's something we would take a close look at."

Each of these examples demonstrates that my research activities sometimes served not merely to record the decisions that people were making but to shape them. I liked to think that when this happened, it wasn't because I was introducing a completely new element into the community. Rather, through my presence as an outsider, the questions I asked and the writings I shared, I was nudging closer to the surface issues or thoughts that already had some limited currency in the minds of some of my informants. Even the case study, then, became part of the social milieu I was studying.

9

Which Way Forward?

I concluded that what the leaders and operators of youth and recreational programs—and the children and families in the case study community needed most of all was a breakthrough in their thinking about the meaning of inclusion. The current thinking patterns were in evidence in nearly all the arenas I investigated. Gretchen, the volunteer leader of the Junior Girl Scout troop, told me that there was no need for any additional modifications in the routines or activities (aside from having a sign language interpreter present) because Jennifer was a "bright child" who could do anything the other girls could do. At the Boys and Girls Club in Brewster, a member of the staff described how he would reply to questions from other youth about Artie's way of speaking or behaving: "He has a disability, and we would appreciate if you would look over that and treat him as a normal person." Sarah, an area consultant for the Girl Scouts, cogitated on what she had learned by being around Lindy: "The main thing I got out of it was that they treated her like she was normal, that's the one thing that sticks in my mind. And that's always what I've tried to do." Two men I interviewed told me of a local boy they knew who had grown up with congenitally malformed hands. Each recalled his ability to shoot with great accuracy in basketball, and both informants emphasized that he was treated just like anyone else, neither expecting nor receiving any special favors.

Remembering the many generations in which youth with disabilities were excluded and stigmatized, each of these statements can be heard as a magnificent tribute to the progress that has been made in the previous two decades. The statements expose a belief in the dignity of every child and a recognition that the right to full participation in the enterprise at hand, whether it be a scout troop, a sports team, a drop-in center, or a pick-up game, is not diminished by one's special need or disability.

INCLUSION AS NONDISCRIMINATION: AN OVERLY NARROW VIEW

Each of the statements, however, also illustrates that the understanding of what it means to include children with disabilities in programs enjoyed by their peers is too narrowly limited. The successful participation of children with special needs often requires peers and leaders to do more than "look over" the fact that someone has a disability, or treat her as if she were "normal." It may require reviewing and revising the way activities and routines have been previously conceived and organized, changing the rules, or introducing new elements into the environment. And this is true, regardless of whether a particular child is viewed as "bright," or as having learning or emotional problems or developmental disabilities.

When Drew, the program director for the Park and Recreation Department, explained that he took a personal hand in selecting coaches for children he knew had special needs, he told me that he would prefer not to be quoted. He clearly believed that such individualized treatment might be viewed as a form of unacceptable discrimination. I never heard anyone else articulate the same point quite so plainly, but I came to believe that it captured well the meaning of inclusion, as understood by program operators, volunteer leaders, and most of the parents as well. Inclusion to them meant first and foremost that children with disabilities should not suffer discrimination.

The federal laws that prohibited discrimination on the basis of disability (principally, Section 504 of the Rehabilitation Act of 1973 and the Americans with Disabilities Act of 1990) were clear and explicit about the meaning of nondiscrimination. They required that organizations and programs make "reasonable accommodations" and "readily achievable modifications" to enable the successful participation of patrons with disabilities. Yet I found that the operators of programs for youth in Wabash and Brewster had not comprehended this. Instead, they had taken to heart what one might call a layman's definition: To include a child with a disability meant not to discriminate. To discriminate was to treat someone differently. To treat someone differently was wrong.

This conception of inclusion as nondiscrimination in its narrow sense seemed to require that they welcome children with disabilities into their groups—and then treat them as if they had no disabilities. Nondiscrimination (and therefore inclusion) did not extend, ordinarily, to modifying programs or activities to accommodate individual needs. Nor did it encompass deliberately facilitating social interaction between the child with special needs and the other participants. This way of thinking, I believe, blocked some program leaders from taking even small steps that would have greatly enhanced the participation of children with disabilities in their activities.

WHAT WOULD ENSUE FROM A BROADER VIEW OF INCLUSION?

Twelve-year-old Jennifer was able to participate with some success in the Junior Girl Scout troop, with her mother or older sister providing sign language interpretation. But without any modifications other than sign language interpretation to accommodate her individual needs, it was apparent to me that Jennifer was left out or bored during parts of every meeting. It did not surprise me at all when, during my interview with her, she expressed her exasperation with the amount of "talking and talking and talking" that took place. I had seen her take extended bathroom breaks, ask for a drink of water, or begin signing and vocalizing whispered sounds to her sister or mother to break the tedium of group discussions.

Toward the end of my interview with Jennifer and her sister Laurie, I told Jennifer that I had an idea and wanted her opinion. I had printed on a card the typical agenda for a troop meeting, numbered from one to six, as follows:

1. Colors (flag ceremony)
2. Business, collect money
3. Discussion of next social event
4. Craft project: making ornaments
5. Play a circle game
6. Snack

I asked her to pretend we were just getting ready to start the meeting, and I was the leader. I was giving her this card so she would know what we would be doing for the whole meeting. She responded that she liked it a lot. I asked Laurie to emphasize that I wasn't looking to be praised for my idea—I just wanted her honest opinion. When Laurie signed this to her, Jennifer became even more animated, saying that it was a very good idea. Laurie then commented that she liked the idea too, and, moreover, she had a portable erasable writing board in the basement, that she could quite easily bring to meetings and use for that purpose. It seemed clear that a modest effort to provide information to Jennifer through visual means would enable her to be much more attuned and considerably less bored.

Tailoring Activities to Individual Capabilities

A clear pattern had also emerged from my observations regarding the types of activities Jennifer loved best: dancing, singing songs that involved body movements or finger snapping, New Games that required getting up and moving around the room, miming, and Halloween games such as bobbing for apples. What did these activities have in common? They did not rely wholly or primarily on oral speech. If the leaders had marginally increased the proportion of the time the troop spent in these sorts of activities, and also provided more visual cues and printed information when oral discussion was on the agenda, the quality of Jennifer's experience would have been greatly enhanced.

Later, while I was completing my writing, I reviewed some of the available resources relevant to situations such as Jennifer's. Carroll (1990, 45) suggests the following for the Girl Scout with hearing impairment: "When the troop or group will be answering questions or discussing a topic, put this information on a chart." Rynders and Schleien (1991, 28) make numerous suggestions for working with a 12-year-old girl with a hearing impairment in a recreational setting, including these: "Use a large easel at meetings and write business items on it with a water color felt-tip pen. Use a dark color. Have a pad and pencil at your meetings for her to write messages to you and vice versa. . . . Make use of the many board and table games that require little or no talking for enjoyable use. Chess, checkers, and various card games are but a few examples of games with modest verbalization demands. . . . Think of other activities that can be enjoyed without talking and therefore require no special adaptations, such as gardening, which offers the pleasures of seeing, moving, touching, and smelling."

In other words, for those who may not think of appropriate adaptations on their own, there are printed resource books available, written in language that is readily comprehensible to the nonspecialist. However, so long as people are committed to the idea that inclusion simply means allowing the child to participate and treating her the same as everyone else, they are not going to develop these plans by their own creative thinking or feel motivated to look for ideas in books. It is their thinking that must change first, to embrace and become comfortable with the concept that inclusion means more than fitting the child into the routines and activities as previously designed for peers without special needs.

Promoting Social Interaction

In the previous chapter, I described my finding that coaches, scout leaders, and recreation supervisors were generally attentive to their specific tasks and instructional goals but seldom if at all to the social interactions or friendship patterns among the participants. If they were to adopt a broader view of inclusion, I would hope that view would lead them to place a greater priority on facilitating social interactions for the child with special needs. For children who are separated from many of their peers during their time in school or who are not viewed as talented in the academic arena, a youth, sports, or recreational program may offer their best chance to have positive social interactions and to make friends.

Staff at the Boys and Girls Club in Brewster, for instance, could have begun the summer with the understanding that it might be more difficult for Artie to make friends than for many other club members, and they could have been on the alert for instances where club members without special needs were relating to him in a positive way. They could have agreed among themselves that it would be acceptable to bend the rules a bit to allow such interactions to take root. Then the 10-year-old who was found hanging around with Artie could have been permitted to stay in the game room as a special guest rather than being reprimanded and sent back to his own age group.

Patsy told me she thought Jennifer would enjoy playing at the YRC but only if she had one or two girlfriends to accompany her. Because the school district bussed Jennifer to Brewster, she didn't know many girls in Wabash. "I'd have to stay there and play with her myself," was Patsy's comment. She might have felt differently about bringing her to the YRC, if she knew that the staff would go out of their way to find Jennifer a companion (and help that companion communicate with her). In fact, Greg talked to me about his commitment to help any child that arrived without a friend to find one. But without any outreach to the families of children with disabilities, and without any explicit communication that the YRC's commitment to inclusion meant not only welcoming them in the door but facilitating their ability to play and interact with peers, there was no chance that Patsy would bring Jennifer there to play.

Paying more attention to the social interaction patterns of children with special needs would have benefits for participants without disabilities as well. It would not hurt the typically developing youngsters at all to have their leaders, supervisors, and mentors watching out to see if someone was lonely, isolated, getting into conflicts frequently, or having a hard time making friends. The supervisors and leaders might also find that by investing energy in facilitating positive social relationships at an earlier point in time, they would have less need to address major discipline problems later on. But we must acknowledge that time spent addressing the peer relationship problems of an individual youth requires time taken away from teaching basketball or working on a patch or a merit badge. We cannot expect recreation supervisors or youth program leaders to do this unless the organizations that recruit and train them have given a clear message that this is an essential part of their role and mission.

Honestly Acknowledging Differences and Disabilities

I was present when several new girls joined Jennifer's Junior Girl Scout troop. They sat around a table and introduced themselves to one another, and when it was Jennifer's turn, she made some whispered sounds, which were not easily intelligible. Translating for her, Gretchen said, "This is Jennifer." No one, then or subsequently, pointed out to the new girls that Jennifer was deaf or suggested ways of communicating with her, such as learning some signs, making gestures, or writing back-and-forth on a note pad. Each troop member was left to make her own observations and draw her own conclusions. One conclusion I would guess they all drew was that Jennifer's deafness was not something to be inquired about or explicitly made a subject of conversation.

This was unfortunate. These girls could not talk with Jennifer as they talked with one another, and they needed help in figuring out how to become friends with her. Moreover, they were at an age when they were keenly aware of individual differences in appearance and development. I listened to one impassioned discussion (in my field notes, I called it an "explosion of talk") regarding which girls in the troop or among their school friends had glasses or were about to get them, and which ones had braces, retainers, or expanders for their teeth. Without permission or encouragement to focus on Jennifer's differences, they kept whatever questions they had to themselves. I did not see any of them make any special efforts to befriend Jennifer or find ways to interact with her.

This was in contrast to what I saw in the Brownie troop in which La-Toya and Erica participated. The troop conducted two meetings at La-Toya's home, and girls got a chance to explore her wheelchair, her alternative communication device, her specialized equipment (such as the lift that lowered her into the bath), and her adapted toys. There was ongoing interest in the way she selected phrases from her Liberator, and no one seemed shy about commenting on the way she communicated with her device. This open recognition of her disabilities did not stigmatize LaToya or separate her from her peers. Rather, it made her differences, which were visible and conspicuous, more understandable. It removed some of the mystery created by the use of paraphernalia and made her more accessible as a person. This is what I thought would have also resulted from a more public recognition of Jennifer's deafness, combined with a discussion about how the other troop members and Jennifer could best communicate with one another. I am not suggesting that this would apply to all special needs and all age levels. For instance, Carlton's teammates did not recognize that he had a disability, and there would have been no benefit to draw attention to it.

In a previous chapter, I described three dimensions of inclusive practice, referred to as curriculum infusion, social inclusion, and learning inclusion (Ferguson, Meyer, Jeanchild, Juniper, and Zingo 1992). Curriculum infusion means making information about disabilities available. Taking the girls to LaToya's house to become familiar with her equipment and toys was a wonderful and useful example of curriculum infusion. Social inclusion means developing a process by which other children could have social interaction with a peer with a disability. This is what I thought was missing in Jennifer's situation. It was apparent that the mere presence of a child with a disability, absent a more conscientious focus on how to support and enhance her participation, did not bring about a fully inclusive experience.

Widening Options for All Participants

It would be of great benefit to children with disabilities if program leaders spent more time thinking about how to facilitate individual children's participation. But the need to tailor accommodations for specific individuals could also be reduced by widening the range of activities available in any given arena.

When Lucy and Celeste brought some extra games and materials to the McDonald's Play Land, as described in an earlier chapter, so that the most physically active girls in their Brownie troop could be offered some quieting-down time, they did not foresee that this expansion of the repertoire would also meet the specific interests and needs of Ariana, their nonambulatory child. It gave her, it turned out, an option that allowed her to get out of her wheelchair and sit on the floor all evening. At any given time, they said that several other girls were also doing the more quiet activities. The wider range of options, although not conceived with her in mind, made it unnecessary to tailor any further modifications to meet her needs.

That insight resonated with what Greg and his staff at the YRC told me, as I described in an earlier chapter: On the occasions when they made available crafts or other options that were less athletically oriented than basketball, they drew a surprisingly large participation from their members. They also found that the gender mix was more nearly equal. I confirmed through conversations and observations that there was a desire on the part of many children for more variety of activity. Billy Walls, who lived in subsidized housing with his nonambulatory brother Skipper, said he used to go every day to the YRC, but stopped going much because he got bored with it. I met girls at the YRC who seemed rowdy and full of physical energy but who calmed down quickly when given a chance to sit and play cards. On the rare occasions when Greg brought out the roller skates and told everyone to put the basketballs away, there was great excitement. When the options were expanded, it improved the chances that each child could find something to match his or her individual abilities, needs, personality, and interests. If more choices were routinely available, then the task of designing or modifying activities for members with special needs would be reduced to a minimum, or made unnecessary.

Increasing Opportunities for Leaders to Share Ideas

When I attended a meeting of Girl Scout leaders from Wabash and nearby towns, I asked those gathered if they had worked with any girls with special needs, and nearly half said yes. When I asked if they had ever had a chance to discuss their experiences with other leaders, they all said no. They agreed that it would be useful for the local council or service unit to sponsor such a discussion.

I also queried them as to what other methods of support might be useful in making their troops more hospitable to girls with disabilities. Someone suggested that in their newsletter, they should put in a reminder notice that the Focus on Ability Task Force could called if anyone needed advice about responding to a troop member with special needs. Another suggested the newsletter could list the names and phone numbers of individual leaders who were working with girls with disabilities. It seemed to me that all the organizations I observed would have been better off with mechanisms in place to encourage such communication and sharing of experiences.

More Direct and Open Recruitment of Youth with Special Needs

No youth development program or recreational organization in Wabash, not even the Girl Scouts with their Focus on Ability Task Force, conducted active outreach, deliberately seeking to identify youth with special needs and recruit them (or their families) as members of teams, clubs, troops, or groups. Each of them was prepared to accept children with disabilities, to a greater or lesser degree, but in no case were they publicly disseminating this message to the community. Their failure to reach out in a public, proactive way may have led some families of youth with special needs to believe that their children would not be fully welcomed.

MacTavish (1995) reports on a survey and interview study she conducted of 65 families with children with disabilities in a single community. She found that "parents almost invariably expressed concern about the messages—the information—they received from recreation service agencies." She quotes one parent (11) stating that the printed materials she receives from the YMCA and the park department "have that generic statement, something about no one being excluded." But that kind of statement was inadequate to reassure her that they were truly prepared to offer the support needed for a child with significant disabilities.

SPORTS RULES—ARE INCLUSIVE PRACTICES OUT OF BOUNDS?

I referred in an earlier chapter to a discussion I heard among baseball coaches in the WPRD. They were debating the pros and cons of a rule that had recently been changed. "How can you change a rule at the end of the game?" one coach wanted to know. "In college basketball," Drew responded, "they stop the clock after every score in the final two minutes. So, yes, if you want to, you can change the rules for one part of the game." He went even further than that, saying that they could tinker with the rules in any manner they wanted, "if we think it meets the needs of the players."

Casey Martin Revisited: What Lessons Might We Draw?

Casey Martin's legal battle with the PGA stands as a further reminder that rules, whether applied to a park and recreation league or a professional sport, are not fixed for centuries but are part of a dynamic process. The chain of events that led to Martin's litigation against the PGA began with the promulgation of a new rule prohibiting the use of a motorized cart during the final stage of a qualifying tournament, even though such carts were permissible during two earlier stages. The rules that had prevailed just one year earlier, in 1996, allowed the carts in all three stages of the tournament. The changes in rules from one year to the next and the fact that rules could vary from one stage to another within a single tournament make it clear that the concept of rule modification was not foreign to professional sports. As Drew reminded his volunteer coaches, such modifications were not unknown in college sports either. Apparently, discussions about rule changes and rule modification do take place within a variety of bodies responsible for governing sports. Prior to the passage of the ADA, however, it was apparently assumed that the needs of athletes with disabilities should not be considered a legitimate basis for triggering discussions of rule changes or rule modifications in sport.

When the federal magistrate ordered the PGA to allow Casey Martin to use a cart during the final stage of the PGA Qualifying Tournament, the PGA made an interesting decision: They announced that all competitors would be allowed to use motorized carts. Out of 168 golfers, observers counted between 10 and 20 who took up the offer (Steve Harrison, "Disabled Pro Golfer Fights No-Cart Rule," *Washington Post*, 10 December 1997, A-14). From this experience, we may draw two important inferences. First, the individual accommodation requested by Martin was not viewed as an important advantage by the vast majority of golfers. Second, an accommodation requested by a participant with a disability turned out to be of apparent benefit to some other athletes, even though they had no disabilities.

It seems to me that allowing this particular modification to anyone who wanted it neither threatened the integrity of the game nor skewed the competition. I agree with Tom Sullivan, writing in *Newsweek* (1998, 16): "So make it easy. Remove the restriction on the use of carts altogether. Don't make Casey Martin an exception: make him a standard."

I stated earlier that whenever a wider range of options became available for participants of all abilities, the need for individualized modifications for those who had disabilities was reduced. Access to a motorized cart on the golf course seems to be one more illlustration of that supposition. Leaders of youth programs of many varieties would do well to be guided by Sullivan's comments. The introduction of alternative ways of participating, whether in hitting a ball or earning a martial arts belt, does not prevent anyone else from continuing to participate in a more traditional manner. But it does open up new opportunities for fun, challenge, and achieving mastery to many who would otherwise be left on the sidelines.

An Empirical Study of Rule Modification in Team Sports

A study was published in 1994 that examined the impact of rule and procedure modifications introduced for a 12-year-old child with significant speech, mobility, and physical impairments in a park district team sports program. Bernabe and Block's (1994) study described the inclusion of "Katie" in a fast-pitch girls' softball league.

An initial set of recommended rule changes were developed by the two researchers, together with Katie's parents. Then these ideas were presented to all the league's volunteer coaches at a preseason meeting. The coaches added their own suggestions, modified those presented, and were given final say on the rule changes. The researchers then surveyed the players in the league to learn how they would react if someone of Katie's description were to play (but keeping her identity unknown) and were to have the benefit of certain rule changes. They asked about each of five possible rule changes and found approval ("yes" or "probably yes") ranging from 80 percent who accepted that she could hit from a tee instead of a pitched ball to 98 percent who accepted that someone could assist her when she played in the field.

Among the rule modifications the coaches adopted were the assignment of Katie only to centerfield (where the leftfielder or rightfielder could back her up), a limit on opposing team's runners to advancing only two bases when Katie handled balls in centerfield, shortening of the distance to first base when Katie came to bat, and letting her hit from a tee (with a limit of three swings) instead of a pitched ball.

The adaptations were judged successful by the authors for a number of reasons. These included the absence of negative feedback from coaches, the fact that games took no longer to play with Katie participating, and the gains she made in batting skill and on-base percentage as the season progressed. Also, the team's won/lost record was about the same in the games she played and in several games she missed.

Like Carlton in the WPRD tee-ball league, Katie missed half of her team's games—7 out of 15—due to illness or vacation. The authors do not comment in the published article on whether these absences in any way undercut the progress they saw her make in improving her skills and becoming familiar with the protocols of the game. However, one of the researchers told me that she not only missed half the games but also about half the practices, and there was no question that she could have made even more progress if she had been able to attend with greater regularity.[1] He also agreed that, given the medical and therapy appointments and other obligations of players with disabilities, coaches should not be surprised if team members with significant disabilities have a hard time maintaining consistent attendance.

What If He Drives in the Winning Run?

As a contribution to my research, Drew clipped from one of the publications he regularly read an article relating to the prevention of injuries in competitive softball leagues. It conveyed the idea that anyone pushing for a kinder, gentler approach to competitive sports (and not just in Wabash) was up against a riptide that pulled from the opposite direction. I took this lesson to be his intention in sharing the story with me.

The article described the efforts of an organization called the Institute for Preventative Sports Medicine, which had conducted research documenting that sliding into base was the number-one cause of softball-related injuries (Cohen 1996, 35). After publishing the research, the institute circulated a proposal to outlaw sliding in the nearby leagues in Ann Arbor, Michigan. "Called 'communists' and worse by some of the more traditionalist elements in the Ann Arbor softball community, the group abandoned that idea."

Not willing to give up on injury prevention, the institute staff next tried to teach local softball players the proper way to slide. "The problem was compliance; very few athletes showed up for their seminars." When last heard from, the researchers had abandoned the prospect of altering either the rules or the behavior of the players. Instead, they were "testing the effectiveness of safety-release bases."

Sitting at the counter of a Wabash diner, I asked Drew what he would say if someone suggested that adaptations such as those devised for Katie in the Bernabe and Block (1994) study be made for a child with disabilities in one of the WPRD leagues. He was cautious about responding to a hypothetical situation, and after a long pause, responded instead with a series of questions.

What if you had a player like Carlton, and he was playing in a player-pitched league, but you brought out a tee when it was his turn to hit? Would that be a good modification? Would that work? At what point does the kid appreciate you doing this for him? Or would it just embarrass him?

And then the next question that comes up is, if, while hitting off the tee, he hits a home run and that allows the team to win the game. Should it count?

Schleien and Ray (1988, 11) stated that "general recreation staff who were previously led to believe that they did not possess the expertise to work effectively with disabled people may question their own abilities to conduct integrated programs." Drew brought research and practice together with his final comment. After quietly posing his series of questions, he said plaintively, "I didn't get any training on this kind of thing."

Notes

INTRODUCTION

1. This information is from a telephone conversation with Geoffrey's mother, Robin Shultz, on September 6, 1996.

2. I learned this from a telephone conversation on March 30, 1999, with Eve Hill, the executive director of the Western Law Center for Disability Rights in Los Angeles, the office that represented Geoffrey Shultz and his family.

3. On October 25, 1999, upon finishing the last match of his second year on the Nike Tour, Martin had accrued the fourteenth highest winnings ($122, 742) on the tour, and thus qualified to play the following season in the PGA Tour (Bill Fields, "Casey Martin earns a spot on PGA Tour," *New York Times*, 25 October 1999, sec. C, p. 3) A decision on the PGA's appeal against his right to use a motorized cart as an accommodation under the ADA was expected no later than April 2000 from the U.S. Court of Appeals for the Ninth Circuit.

4. This information was provided to me in a telephone conversation with Robin Shultz, September 1, 1996.

5. Jeffrey Tolley's poems became known to me because they were first published in *NC Crossroads*, vol. 2, no. 2, April 1998, a publication of the North Carolina Humanities Council. Subsequently, I spoke with Susan Davis by telephone on February 8, 1999, and she helped me to obtain consent from the author.

CHAPTER 1

1. Unified Sports, an inclusive initiative of Special Olympics in which teams were made up of half members with and half without mental disabilities, had not yet come to Brewster as of 1997, although they were "trying to get it going" in softball.

CHAPTER 3

1. Just exactly how much population Wabash lost at the time its major employer closed shop—and how much it had regained due to subsequent efforts at economic development—was a subject of contention. The Regional Planning Commission of the county in which Wabash is located featured an article in its "State of the County Population Supplement," in May 1996, examining a variety of estimates of the population of Wabash (Malhotra, 1996).

2. The figure I was given for a full Girl Scout uniform was approximately $60.

3. This number does not include two children who died prior to the beginning of the study: Lindy and Peter (Rosemary's son).

4. Even the diagnosis that her parents finally received and accepted was under renewed scrutiny at the time I interviewed them. The onset of her illness did not follow the usual course of Guillain-Barre' syndrome. However, for any of the possible alternative explanations of her symptoms, "the interventions would be the same," according to her father, so the accuracy of the diagnosis was no longer a central issue to the family.

5. I obtained the school district data in this and following paragraphs in personal correspondence dated May 17, 1996, from an administrator for the school district I have fictionalized as Wabash.

6. I did not collect comparable data from the high school administration, because my focus was on the recreational and youth development activities of elementary-and junior high–aged youth with special needs. (I did, nevertheless, interview two high school students with disabilities that came to my attention.)

CHAPTER 4

1. Cerebral palsy is a disorder of muscle control or coordination resulting from injury to the brain during fetal, perinatal, and early childhood stages of development. There may be associated problems with intellectual, visual, or other functions (Healy 1983).

2. This statement is excerpted from a one-page mission statement of the Youth Baseball Athletic League that was being circulated in 1996–97 and

signed by its founder and commissioner, Chuck Alley. The organization's offices were located in Palo Alto, California.

CHAPTER 5

1. Greg, the YRC director, took a Polaroid photograph of the napping boy, saying with a smile to the children nearby, "We'll show his mother a picture of what he looks like when he's being good!"

2. The source of this information is a newspaper article headlined, "Youth center programs have broad appeal," published on June 3, 1996, on page one of the weekly newspaper in the community I have called Wabash.

3. Artie's sister Karen gave me an explanation of the differences between the Boys and Girls Club in Brewster and another one she used to attend in Virginia. I found it wonderfully reflective of her developmental stage (nine years old): "There's two things different. In the other one, you don't stay with your age group." (Pause.) "And there's no upstairs."

CHAPTER 6

1. Judith B. Erickson, scholar and librarian of the Indiana Youth Institute, provided the background information about the Order of the American Boy and access to her files, on November 1, 1995.

2. The Americans with Disabilities Act, passed in 1990 a few years after the events described in Rosemary's story, might have produced a different ending to the tale. The law stipulates that when separate activities for those with disabilities are offered by any organization considered to be a public accommodation (a designation that would cover the Boy Scouts), it must be an option. Individuals with disabilities as defined by the law who prefer to attend the regular activities and can do so successfully with the help of readily achievable modifications must be allowed to do so.

3. *The Exceptional Parent* (Klein 1996) reported that Adam Thal, age 22, was on the way to becoming one of the first young men with mental retardation to receive the organization's highest award, the Eagle Scout. He had joined his troop in the Washington, D.C., area, in 1989—just two years after Rosemary's unfortunate experience at the Tiger Cub picnic in Wabash. Obviously, the change from separate units for those with special needs to more inclusive programming was taking place unevenly across the country within the Boy Scouts as within other youth programs.

4. For older girls (Cadette and Senior Girl Scouts), the Focus on Ability Task Force organized visits to facilities on the campus of the state university in Brewster, such as the rehabilitation units for students with special physical, sensory, and learning needs, and a special dormitory for students with severe physical disabilities.

CHAPTER 7

1. Henry had little memory of his special education experience. He could remember that he saw a speech therapist "for my talking," but not that he also had regular visits with occupational and physical therapists through his kindergarten year.

2. A reference to a routine on Bill Cosby's first comedy recording, an album released when I was in high school.

CHAPTER 9

1. On January 15, 1997, I discussed the research with Martin Block, co-author of the 1994 study, in a telephone conversation.

Selected Bibliography

Arbogast, G., and Lavay, B. 1987. Combining students with different ability levels in games and sports. *Physical Educator* 44: 255–260.

Bernabe, E. A., and Block, M. E. 1994. Modifying rules of a regular girls softball league to facilitate the inclusion of a child with severe disabilities. *Journal of The Association for Persons with Severe Handicaps* 19: 24–31.

Bogdan, R. C., and Biklen, S. K. 1992. *Qualitative research for education.* Boston: Allyn and Bacon.

Bogdan, R., and Kugelmass, J. 1984. Case studies of mainstreaming: A symbolic interactionist approach to special schooling. In *Special education and social interests,* edited by L. Barton and S. Tomlinson. New York: Nichols Publishing Company.

Boy Scouts of America. 1922. *Annual report of the boy scouts of America.* New York: Boy Scouts of America.

Boy Scouts of America. 1923. *Fourteenth annual report of the boy scouts of America.* New York: Boy Scouts of America.

Boy Scouts of America. 1965. *Annual report of the boy scouts of America.* North Brunswick, NJ: Boy Scouts of America.

Boy Scouts of America. 1975. *Understanding cub scouts with disabilities.* Irving, TX: Boy Scouts of America.

Boy Scouts of America. 1994. Fact sheet; scouts with special needs. Available from External Communications, 1325 West Walnut Hill Lane, P.O. Box 152079, Irving, Texas 75015–2079.

Boys Clubs of America. 1985. *Mainstreaming matters: A guide for working with emotionally, physically and learning disabled children.* New York: Boys Clubs of America.

Carnegie Council on Adolescent Development, Carnegie Corporation of New York. 1992. *A matter of time: Risk and opportunity in the non-school hours.* New York: Carnegie Council on Adolescent Development.

Carroll, M. E. 1990. *Focus on ability: Serving girls with special needs.* New York: Girl Scouts of the USA.

Chapel Hill Parks and Recreation Department. 1990. Accessibility. Winter/Spring, Chapel Hill Parks and Recreation Department, Chapel Hill, NC.

Cohen, A. 1996. Save situations. *Athletic Business* 20 (80): 33–38.

Cooperative Extension Service of Purdue University. n.d. *A perfect fit/4-H involvement for youth with disabilities, a leader's guide.* W. Lafayette, IN: Purdue University.

Denzin, Norman. 1989. *Interpretive interactionism.* Newbury Park, CA: Sage Publications.

DePauw, Karen P., and Gavron, Susan J. 1995. *Disability and sport.* Champaign, IL: Human Kinetics.

Ferguson, D. L., and Baumgart, D. 1991. Partial participation revisited. *Journal of The Association for Persons with Severe Handicaps* 16: 218–227.

Ferguson, D. L., Meyer, G., Jeanchild, L., Juniper, L., and Zingo, J. 1992. Figuring out what to do with the grownups: How teachers make inclusion "work" for students with disabilities. *Journal of The Association for Persons with Severe Handicaps* 17: 218–226.

Fine, G. A., and Sandstrom, K. L. 1988. *Knowing children: Participant observation with minors.* Newbury Park, CA: Sage Publications.

Fink, D. B. 1988. *School-age children with special needs: What do they do when school is out?* Boston: The Exceptional Parent Press.

Girl Scouts of the USA. 1994. Focus on ability: Reaching out to girls and adults with disabilities. *Membership News and Views* (May). New York: Girl Scouts of the USA.

Graue, M. E., and Walsh, D. J. 1995. Children in context: Interpreting the here and now of children's lives. In *Qualitative research in early childhood settings,* edited by J. A. Hatch. Westport, CT: Praeger.

Healy, A. 1983. Cerebral palsy. In *Medical aspects of developmental disabilities in children birth to three,* edited by J. A. Blackman. Gaithersburg, MD: Aspen Publisher.

Johnson, A., and Johnson, O. R. 1990. Quality into quantity: On the measurement potential of ethographic fieldnotes. In *Fieldnotes, the mak-*

ings of anthropology, edited by R. Sanjek. Ithaca: Cornell University Press.

Klein, S. D. 1996. 25 role models for the next 25 years. *Exceptional Parent*, June, 48–59.

Krebs, P., and Cloutier, G. 1992. Unified sports: I've seen the future. *Palaestra* 8 (2): 42–44.

Lincoln, Y. S., and Guba, E. G. 1985. *Naturalistic inquiry*. Newbury Park, CA: Sage Publications.

MacTavish, J. 1995. Why is a family focus imperative to inclusive recreation? In *Powerful partnerships: Parents and professionals building inclusive recreation programs together*, edited by S. J. Schleien, J. E. Rynders, L. A. Heyne, and C.E.S. Tabourne. Minneapolis: The College of Education, University of Minnesota.

MacTavish, J. B. 1994. Recreation in families that include children with developmental disabilities: Nature, benefits, and constraints. Ph.D. diss., University of Minnesota.

Malhotra, U. 1996. State of the county population supplement. Urbana, IL: Champaign County Regional Planning Commission.

Miles, M. B., and Huberman, A. M. 1984. Drawing valid meaning from qualitative data: Toward a shared craft. *Educational Researcher* 13 (5): 20–30.

Miles, M. B., and Huberman, A. M. 1994. *Qualitative data analysis*. Thousand Oaks, CA: Sage Publications.

Mishler, E. G. 1986. *Research interviewing*. Cambridge: Harvard University Press.

Moon, M. S. 1994. The case for inclusive school and community recreation. In *Making school and community recreation run for everyone: Places and ways to integrate*, edited by M. S. Moon. Baltimore: Paul H. Brookes Publishing Company.

Moon, M. S., Hart, D., Komissar, C., and Friedlander, R. 1995. Making sports and recreation activities accessible: Assistive technology and other accommodation strategies. In *Assistive technology*, edited by K. Flippo, K. Inge, and M. Barcus. Baltimore: Paul H. Brookes Publishing Company.

National Collaboration for Youth. 1990. Making the grade: A report card on American youth—report on the nationwide project. Washington, DC: National Collaboration for Youth.

Peshkin, A. 1988. In search of subjectivity—one's own. *Educational Researcher* 17 (7): 17–22.

Richardson, D., Wilson, B., Wetherald, L., and Peters, J. 1987. Mainstreaming initiative: An innovative approach to recreation and leisure services in a community setting. *Therapeutic Recreation Journal* (second quarter): 9–19.

Rynders, J. E., and Schleien, S. J. 1991. *Together successfully: Creating recreational and educational programs that integrate people with and without disabilities.* Arlington, TX: Association for Retarded Citizens of the United States; National Office of 4-H and Youth Development; Research and Training Center on Community Living, University of Minnesota, Institute on Community Integration (UAP), University of Minnesota.

Sable, J. 1992. Collaborating to create an integrated camping program: Design and evaluation. *Therapeutic Recreation Journal* 26: 38–48.

Salzman, M. 1987. *Iron and silk.* New York: Vintage Books.

Sanjek, R., ed. 1990. *Fieldnotes; The makings of anthropology.* Ithaca: Cornell University Press.

Schleien, S. J., McAvoy, L. H., Lais, G. J., and Rynders, J.E. 1993. *Integrated outdoor education and adventure programs.* Champaign, IL: Sagamore Publishing.

Schleien, S. J., and Ray, M. T. 1988. *Community recreation and persons with disabilities: Strategies for integration.* Baltimore: Paul H. Brookes Publishing Company.

Schleien, S. J., Tabourne, C.E.S., and Dart, P. C. 1995. Why is inclusive recreation important? In *Powerful partnerships: Parents and professionals building inclusive recreation programs together,* edited by S. J. Schleien, J. E. Rynders, L. A. Heyne, and C.E.S. Tabourne. Minneapolis: The College of Education, University of Minnesota.

Schleien, S. J., and Werder, J. K. 1985. Perceived responsibilities of special recreation services in Minnesota. *Therapeutic Recreation Journal* 19 (3): 51–62.

Shapiro, J. P. 1991. Keeping pace. *U.S. News and World Report,* 5 August, 11.

Stake, R. E. 1978. The case study method in social inquiry. *Educational Researcher* 7: 5–8.

Stake, R. E. 1994. Case studies. In *Handbook of qualitative research,* edited by N.K. Denzin and E. S. Lincoln. Thousand Oaks, CA: Sage Publications.

Stake, R. E. 1995. *The art of case study research.* Thousand Oaks, CA: Sage Publications.

Stake, R. E., Bresler, L., and Mabry, L. 1991. *Custom and cherishing: The arts in elementary schools.* Urbana: National Arts Research Center, University of Illinois.

Staub, D., Schwartz, I. S., Gallucci, C., and Peck, C. A. 1994. Four portraits of friendship at an inclusive school. *Journal of The Association for Persons with Severe Handicaps* 19: 314–325.

Tabourne, C.E.S., Schleien, S. J., and Dart, P. C. 1995. To play or not to play? A history of recreation in America. In *Powerful partnerships:*

Parents and professionals building inclusive recreation programs together, edited by S. J. Schleien, J. E. Rynders, L. A. Heyne, and C.E.S. Tabourne. Minneapolis: The College of Education, University of Minnesota.

U.S. Department of Education. 1997. *Nineteenth annual report to Congress on the implementation of the Individuals with Disabilities Education Act.*

Van Manen, M. 1990. *Researching lived experience.* London, Ontario, Canada: State University of New York Press.

Vinland Inclusion Project (1995). *Access to opportunities/How to include people of all abilities in community programs.* Available from Vinland Center, 3675 Iduhapi Rd., P.O. Box 308, Loretto, MN 55357.

Walker, P. 1988. Supporting children in integrated recreation. *The Association for Persons with Severe Handicaps Newsletter*, January, 4–5.

Walker, P. 1990. Supports for children and teens with severe disabilities in integrated recreation/leisure activities. In *Resources on integrated recreation/leisure opportunities for children and teens with developmental disabilities*, edited by P. Walker. Syracuse, NY: Center on Human Policy, Syracuse University.

Walker, P. 1994. Promoting inclusive recreation and leisure options for adults. In *Making school and community recreation run for everyone: Places and ways to integrate*, edited by M. S. Moon. Baltimore: Paul H. Brookes Publishing Company.

Walker, P., and Edinger, B. 1988. The kid from cabin 17. *Camping Magazine*, May, 18–21.

Walsh, D. J., Tobin, J. T., and Graue, M. E. 1993. The interpretive voice: Qualitative research in early childhood education. In *Handbook of research on the education of young children*, edited by B. Spodek. New York: MacMillan Publishing Company.

Weiss, L., Rynders, J. E., and Schleien, S. J. 1995. Working together for programs of quality. In *Powerful partnerships; parents and professionals building inclusive recreation programs together*, edited by S. J. Schleien, J. E. Rynders, L. A. Heyne, and C.E.S. Tabourne. Minneapolis: The College of Education, University of Minnesota.

Wolff, G. 1979. *The duke of deception.* New York: Random House.

Young Men's Christian Associations of the United States of America. 1980. *Mainstreaming (Books 1, 2, and 3).* Longview, WA: Project MAY of the National Council of the YMCA.

Index

About the Author

DALE BORMAN FINK is a freelance consultant, author, and researcher. Dr. Fink is recognized as one of the nation's leading authorities on the inclusion of children with disabilities in after-school child care programs. His book, *School-Age Children With Special Needs: What Do They Do When School Is Out?*, is the key source on this topic. He has been a featured speaker at conferences across the United States as well as in Canada and Australia.

ISBN 0-275-96565-1

90000>

EAN

9 780275 965655

HARDCOVER BAR CODE

DATE DUE

MAR			
NOV 1 5 2001			
APR 1 8 2002			
NOV 1 1 2002			
			Printed in USA